CREATING THERAPEUTIC ACTIVITY PLANS IN LONG TERM CARE FACILITIES: THE BASIC PRINCIPLES

JAMES W. RAMAGE, PH. D.

Bloomington, IN 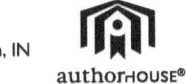 Milton Keynes, UK

authorHOUSE®

AuthorHouse™
1663 Liberty Drive, Suite 200
Bloomington, IN 47403
www.authorhouse.com
Phone: 1-800-839-8640

AuthorHouse™ UK Ltd.
500 Avebury Boulevard
Central Milton Keynes, MK9 2BE
www.authorhouse.co.uk
Phone: 08001974150

First published by AuthorHouse   8/24/2006

ISBN: 1-4208-8003-9 (sc)

Printed in the United States of America
Bloomington, Indiana

This book is printed on acid-free paper.

IN MEMORY OF

Jennie Moore, a unique soul who lived briefly among us sharing those gifts of the spirits – service, humbleness, humility, forgiveness, creativity, clarity and love. She was an example of a soul that lived life with purpose, fully whole, empowered and inwardly secure. She was that point of light between energy and matter, a soul, comfortable with her spirituality, in harmony with those creative, life-giving and wholesome forces of the universe. Her vitality, boundless energy and thirst for life will be remembered but underscores the critical need for mankind to rethink the whole notion of the human process.

Contents

DEDICATION

To my children: Deborah, James II, and Elizabeth (Beth); and to my Grandchildren: Bobby, Hunter and Jordon; who make my life worthwhile, I dedicate the following thoughts:

SOMEDAY

Some day, when I am never old
That only happens to someone else
I hope to sing, just to sing
To be happy, just to be happy.

Someday, when I am never old
That only happens to someone else
I hope, someone will sit with me
Just to sit with me.

Some day, when I am never old
That only happens to someone else
I hope, someone will listen to me
Just to listen to me.

Some day, when I am never old
That only happens to someone else
I hope someone will talk to me
Just to talk to me.

Some day, when I am never old
That only happens to someone else
I hope someone will share with me
Just to share with me.

Some day, when I am never old
That only happens to someone else
I hope to dream, just to dream
To feel the wind beneath my wings.

Some day, when I am never old
That only happens to someone else
I hope to fly, just fly
To catch a falling star, just to catch a star.

Some day, when I am never old
That only happens to someone else
I hope to work, just to work
To express myself, just to express myself.

Some day, when I am never old

That only happens to someone else

I hope to search, just to search

To touch the Hand of God, Just to touch the Hand of God.

SOME DAY WHEN I AM NEVER OLD - - - - - - - - - - -

OLD – AGE; QUOTES FROM THE ANCIENTS

To know how to grow old is the Master work of wisdom, and one of the most difficult chapters in the art of living. Amiel., Philosopher. (1874).

Every thought is afterthought. Arendt., Philosopher. (1977).

Old men are twice children. Aristophanes. Poet. (423 B.C.)

Man is as old as his connective tissues. Bogomoletz, Physician. (1946).

A man is as old as his arteries. Metchnikoff. Scientist. (1845 – 1916).

Youth is a blunder; manhood a struggle; old age a regret. Disraeli. Writer. (1844).

Old age is more to be feared than death. Juveualis. Poet. (140 A.D.).

A man is sane morally at 30; rich mentally at 40; wise spiritually at 50 – or never – or well. Osler. (1905).

When men grow virtuous in their old age, they only make a sacrifice to God of the devil's leavings. Pope. Poet. (1727).

Few people know how to be old. Rochhefoocaold. Writer. (1664).

Those who cannot remember the past are condemned to repeat it. Santayana. Philosopher. (1906).

Nothing is less worthy of honor than an old man who has no other evidence of having lived long except his age. Seneca. (4 B.C. – 65 A.D.).

Old age should burn and rave at the close of day. Thomas, (1953).

Every man desires to live long, but no man would be old. Swift. Educator. (1706).

No one is old until they think old. Leon Trotsky. (1935).

Old age is the most unexpected of all the things that can happen to a man. Leon Trotsky.

That is the great fallacy, the wisdom of old men, they do not grow wise, they grow careful. Hemingway. (1929).

ACKNOWLEDGEMENTS

I want to extend my appreciation to the many individuals who were instrumental in developing this book. First, of course, are the untold number of nursing home residents with whom I have worked over the past thirty years. This experience has afforded me the opportunity to glance briefly into their mystical and nostalgic world, and to develop a feeling of intimacy and kinship with them as we confronted together their dreaded "old timers disease". The journey has expanded my knowledge, deepened my compassion and has been a wonderful, exciting, rewarding experience, and a professional challenge.

Although these elderly men and women have generally been cognitively impaired, physically frail, and in poor health, they never cease to amaze me with their knowledge, abilities, and diversity. Each shared with me pictures of themselves when they were young, attractive, or not so attractive; each had a story(s) to tell and did so with me unselfishly. They were, for the most part, great teachers and on more than one occasion I found myself in the role of a student, and benefited from their wisdom. I was enriched by their strength, sincerity, belief system(s), values, loyalty, outlook on life and their dedication to their God, family and country. I thank each and every one of them for these experiences.

And to the numerous caregivers with whom I have worked. I thank them. There were times when we should have done things differently but didn't, although our intentions were good. However, we were big enough to admit our mistakes, learn from them and move on by concentrating on the many things that we had done well. It seems it was always a daily struggle to make care giving decisions trying to always do a balancing act between what was needed by the resident in our care and what the staff was capable of providing as caregivers to the resident and their families. There were times when the level of stress was so severe that we had to hug a friend, give ourselves a good talking to, or have a good therapeutic cry. To these dedicated caregivers, I give my heartfelt thanks and apologize for not being able to do more to assist.

In reflection, I want to thank and express my sincere appreciation to all nursing home personnel both individually and collectively who tolerated my early presentations on the subjects of "the interdisciplinary team", "the team approach" and "continuity of care". I appreciate their efforts to comprehend how such a social invention could possibly be of any importance in providing more effective help to residents in their care.

And to those brave souls who labored in unchartered waters, during these early years, as activity workers I would like to thank them for their patience and understanding. They not only tolerated me but also accepted me as one of their own. Not only did they accept me but they took time out of their busy schedule to train me in the art of how to be more effective in my role as a consultant. And, of course, now I know that this simply meant that they trained me to permit them to form their own ideas and reach their own conclusions. When translated, this means I am what I am by the grace of those bright and talented men and women who toiled as activity workers in the trenches doing "God's Work" and doing it well.

I appreciate this opportunity of presenting myself to you in apparent blasphemy of all of what I believe in and feel strongly about. It could be that I am doing it out of concern for myself. It could be that I am doing it out of concern for my profession, my place in society or the environment in which I live. However, regardless of these factors I feel the need to share with you my sense of urgency and deep sense of responsibility for what I do, what you do, what our residents do, and what we as professionals do and why.

Also, I would like to thank all the long-term care facilities to which I have served as consultant over the years. I would especially like to express my appreciation to two "Five Star" Facilities at which I consult. The first facility is Daniel Health Care, Inc. located in Fulton, Mississippi. They offer a comprehensive program of services to the elderly, including an Alzheimer's Unit. Their facility is modern, well designed, well staffed and reflects current philosophy for providing healthcare for the elderly. More specifically, I would like to thank Mr. James C. Holland, Owner and Administrator of the facility for his creative and pro-active management style of the facility. He is a long time friend who has tolerated me in his facility all these years. I thank him for his interest, support, and commitment. Also, I would like to extend my appreciation to Ms. Phyllis Wilburn, Administrator of the facility, for her timely criticism and contributions. In particular, I would like to thank the Social Work Staff: Mrs. Kay Painter and Ms. Stacy North, for their interest and constructive comments. And to the Activity Staff, Ms. Lois Bell and Ms. Tammy Strickland, I wish to thank them for their positive input, interest, hard work and dedication.

The second "Five Star" facility which impresses me is The Windsor Place at Plantation Pointe and Philwood Suites located in Columbus, Mississippi. The facility, as indicated by its traditional southern name, is first class in every sense of the word. They have an excellent program of services which are comprehensive in nature including a Special Care Unit for the Alzheimer's resident and families. I am grateful to Ms. Sherry G. Davis, Administrator of the facility, for her innovative management style, interest and enthusiasm. I also wish to thank Ms. Brenda Forcey, Director of the Alzheimer's Unit for her hard work and timely input. And to the Social Work Staff: Ms. Charlotte Howard, and Ms. Misty Holder for their suggestions and the activity staff: Ms. Naomi Forstner and Ms. Marcia Hill, for their efforts. I appreciate each and every comment given by these caregivers.

And, finally, I wish to thank my wife for her hard work, timely criticisms and input into reading, typing and editing this manuscript. In addition to being my wife, she is my soul mate, my buddy, and my best friend. She is and has always been a trooper.

PREFACE

The author had two goals in preparing this book. First, I attempted to convey some of my excitement about the field of Therapeutic Activities. And, in doing so, I chose to address the issue in the form of a workbook rather than a textbook or novel as I felt this excitement should be construed in a figural rather than a literal sense. While I have not presented "sexy" anecdotes, I have tried to describe what the therapeutic specialist should do, how he or she should approach designing and implementing therapeutic activities, and how they should evaluate them to insure accountability.

Much of the excitement about the field stems from the tremendous diversity of activities the therapeutic activity specialist engages in – the social impact of those activities, and the dynamism of applied research such as developing, implementing and evaluating new clinical procedures and redefining existing or old ones. There are few professions which afford the opportunity to engage in such a variety of activities (clinical practice, teaching, research, and consultation) and at the same time experience the personal satisfaction of helping others. Whether through direct clinical services, teaching, or indirectly through research accomplishments, therapeutic activities is and will continue to be a service oriented profession.

My second goal was to provide an empirical picture of the field as the profession moves from a philosophy of general, leisure – time activities to a clinical one designed with treatment objectives based upon a diagnostic assessment. While clinical intuition and self – appraisal may be valuable sources of information, one must ultimately rely on research to adequately understand behavior and evaluate clinical techniques used for treatment.

Therefore, we as a discipline must endeavor to follow descriptions of the predominant treatment techniques and orientations with up – to – date research reviews. As one critiques research literature, it will quickly become evident that some popular procedures will have ample empirical support while others will not. Some are even contraindicated by the research literature. However, activity personnel should not be overly concerned by this state of affairs – it occurs in every discipline. Instead, he or she should be encouraged by the rapid development and change in the field. Therapeutic Activities is still in its infancy. Therapeutic Activities really only began in the early 1970s and there is much work yet to be done. This is part of the stimulus, for my excitement.

By history we come from recreational programs which when examined present a shallow example of a therapeutic philosophy. We are now charged to turn to one with depth, with meaning, with excitement, with relevance, and with fulfillment for our residents. I suggest a good place, perhaps the only place, to begin is right in your facility, right with the resident, defining who is the resident – he or she, what are the human qualities, the human differences?

Working with the elderly has been a challenge, an education, and a privilege for me. As a geriatric practitioner for over thirty years, I have been enriched by their wisdom and perspective on life. It is with great humility that I will attempt to share with you, the activity specialist and health care provider alike, some of the knowledge and techniques of providing treatment and strategies used when relating to this fantastic group of elderly citizens and residents in our long – term care facilities. I hope we can come together, blend our wisdom, and begin to function as a team, developing goals, objectives, and treatment strategies which reflect our thought, ethical consideration, and compassion, insuring effective treatment and documentation. And, hopefully, we will do so while at the same time being extremely sensitive to the unique conditions, situations, strengths, needs, and challenges of the resident(s) as their individual therapeutic activity plan is written.

And during the process, let's develop a philosophy of personal dignity for ourselves, for our residents, and for their families. Lets begin by assessing their lifestyles, strengths, and needs by combining their activities with their environment, by fitting the environment to the desires and needs of the individual. And then, decide what is and what should be therapeutic recreational activities for the elderly. Tell me as a consultant. Let your residents tell you. Listen, and then listen some more to them. Some and maybe all of them will tell you – "I've made a living all my life and now I want to make a difference." Help me, help him, help her, help the one sitting next to you. Help all of us to understand. It's the difference that counts, and it's the activity in action. It's the team approach and continuity of care at its best.

INTRODUCTION

The purpose of this book is to assist personnel charged with developing and implementing therapeutic activity programs for the elderly residing in long term care facilities. Then, too, it can be helpful to caregivers, in general, who are caring for the elderly in their homes and community. It should be especially useful to those specially designed facilities providing care for residents suffering from Alzheimer's Dementia. Also the material can be used by family and relatives to address those issues associated with Dementia in the elderly such as significant memory loss, communication, practical living skills (ADLs) and an inability to recognize familiar things and objects in the community to name a few.

The contents are intended to be a comprehensive, practical, and no-nonsense "cookbook" type of text which provides answers to questions frequently asked by caregivers providing care for the elderly. And finally, it will hopefully motivate activity personnel working in long-term care facilities to become proactive in implementing activities which adhere to current recreational philosophy, address and meet the criteria of therapeutic programming. These criteria are:

1. All activity plans must have goals and objectives;

2. The objectives must be specifically written for each resident following a comprehensive assessment addressing their individual needs.

3. They must be observable, measurable and time-linked;

4. They must be out-come-oriented;

5. They must emphasize competency;

6. They must be written in a positive language;

7. They must reflect sequential and progressive behavior;

8. They must be realistic;

9. They must be understandable to both staff and resident;

10. They must reflect team input and continuity of care.

Further, this book was compiled to be read and understood by persons with little or no formal training in psychology or behavior modification techniques. It has been written in everyday language. Principles have been deliberately kept to a minimum. They are discussed in simple everyday terminology, and are illustrated using experiences common to everyone. No attempt is made to teach the reader how to talk like a psychotherapist. Instead, emphasis is placed on training the reader to become an effective behavior analyst who is capable of analyzing behavior of the Alzheimer's patient and developing activity programs which are therapeutic in nature, and which will modify or maintain the residents behavior in the direction of normal and/or acceptable behavior. Redundancy, which is annoying to some individuals, is used to facilitate the residents learning.

When purchasing real estate, the buyer should always think about the three L's---Location, Location, Location. When working with the Alzheimer's resident the caregiver should always think about the three B's---Behavior, Behavior, Behavior. As a behavior analyst, the activity specialist should realize that when an Alzheimer's resident is observed and assessed, it is like watching a video of life in reverse. For example, parents teach their children appropriate modes of behavior---how to walk, talk, feed themselves, bathe, use the toilet, and how to behave in public. As they mature into teenagers, parents teach them appropriate manners, self control, and accountability. In this process, all these modes of behavior or skills are stored on nerve cells. However, Alzheimer's disease kills these brain cells and these human skills are lost. Therefore, these dying brain cells cause adult behavior to reverse itself. Over time the symptoms of Alzheimer's disease change and no two residents follow the same path during their illness and the degenerative process.

However, their journey is easier when the activity specialist understands the present and future symptoms of the illness realizing that each state of the illness is one of regression of the resident back to that of a 5 or 10 year old child. Therefore, it is imperative that a thorough comprehensive assessment be done before designing and implementing a therapeutic activity plan. And then, it should be done with the same guarded approach, patience, protection and love with which parents treat their children or grandchildren. It should be done with the realization that the Alzheimer's resident is still a mature person that deserves dignity, respect, and age appropriate activities.

Federal regulations (O.B.R.A.) now mandates that therapeutic activities must be provided for all residents living in long term care facilities. This is especially true for those facilities providing special care and services to the elderly suffering from Alzheimer's disease and their family. In other words, these facilities must now, as required by law, provide therapeutic activities to all residents in long term care facilities. And, further, no one can be excluded from or included in these activity programs as a means of "punishment" for inappropriate behavior. Instead a therapeutic activity must be written and implemented to accommodate the residents special needs. This Federal Legislation requiring therapeutic activities in long term care facilities represents a major change in the focus and philosophy of the professional recreator. It has moved the profession from a model of recreation which focused on play, and leisure-time to a clinical one...that of therapeutic activities.

Then too, this change in philosophy has been significant in that it reflected the maturity of the profession of recreation and sophistication of a field which is unlike any other discipline in its concern for the Alzheimer's resident. And during the process of change the profession has kept its boundaries open to facilitate a healthy cross-fertilization of ideas and concepts generated from within the profession as well as from other disciplines. This change has also resulted in the profession gaining professional respectability and acceptance by other disciplines as being a provider that possesses skills and a knowledge base which is unique in its specialization. As a result, therapeutic activities is proving to be one of the best means of breaking down attitudinal barriers which surround the nursing home, the resident, Alzheimer's dementia, and families trying to cope with the disease and the behavior associated with it.

Developing and writing an individual therapeutic activity plan for the Alzheimer's resident can be a challenge for many activity specialists. For example, the Alzheimer's resident with limited cognitive abilities present two very different problems. First, the activity specialist must determine the residents physical limitations and its effect on his or her ability to participate in the activity. And secondly, develop, write and implement all activity programs using creativity, understanding and patience.

Then, too, these residents suffering from Alzheimer's Disease and other dementias present an entirely different challenge. They cannot knowingly decide if they want to or do not want to participate in an activity because they do not have that mental ability. With memory impaired residents, it is helpful to identify inappropriate behavior when preparing an effective activity plan. In addition, knowing the residents past history and understanding their fears assists all staff members in relating to the resident in a positive meaningful and creative manner. Therefore, the approach to involving a resident in activities must always reflect these differences.

Also, there are those residents who present a psychiatric challenge...
these "unstable" psychiatric residents who have experienced and suffered
from a mental or emotional illness most of their lives and who may or
may not have an overlapping dementia such as Alzheimer's disease. All
of the issues which are addressed with other groups of residents exist in
this situation. These psychiatric residents may be manipulative, fright-
ened, have poor impulse control or suffer from depression with a poor
self image and low self esteem...wherever their illness has taken them
which demands even more special care and understanding on the part
of the activity specialist.

Further, working with the Alzheimer's resident over time is generally always stressful due to the complex nature of the disease and the
physical, mental and emotional needs of the individual. And stress
results in burnout of the provider. Some things that might help would
be administrative support, rotation of staff, avoiding stressful events
when away from facility, use of volunteers, the development of positive relationships with other departments, and maintaining good team
work. Team work is always important in inspiring creativity and in
relieving stress. And having an on-going inservice training program
to explore accepted ways as well as new and innovative means of
guarding against burnout is helpful. It is important to remember that
dealing with the elderly Alzheimer's resident need not be a behavioral
management nightmare. It does, however, require patience along with
a cohesive and consistent effort on the part of team members. The
team should focus on management of behavior rather than on modify-

ing it. Remember, it is the residents inappropriate behavior at home or in the community that usually brings him or her to the facility in the first place and not the disease. Therefore, a team effort is vital to the concept of successful behavior management, and it helps the staff guard against burnout.

The recent Federal Legislation reflects societies concern and desire to establish facilities to provide special care for the elderly suffering from Alzheimer's disease. The need has been well documented. According to the latest research sixty (60) percent of all nursing home residents have some form of dementia at the time of admission severe enough to require psychiatric intervention. Then, too, statistics reveal that more than eighty (80) percent of nursing home residents have a mental or emotional problem so acute as to warrant psychological assistance by a mental health professional. Also the need to develop such facilities was influenced by the magnitude of the disease in society, its complex origin, and the challenges on the family of caregivers. And finally, the movement was driven by both the lay and professional communities which provided widespread support for facilities capable of providing a more comprehensive and individualized, program of services to address the complex nature of problems of residents with Alzheimer's disease.

And, due to the number, severity and complex needs of the Alzheimer's resident, concerns of the family, and demands on direct care staff and caregivers, the activity specialist can bring their area of expertise to bear on the treatment and management of the residents who suffer from Alzheimer's disease. The activity specialist can, as they expand their base of knowledge of individual personality growth and development, develop an awareness of the basic techniques in guidance and counseling serve as a counselor, functioning much as a psychologist or social worker to relieve much of the anger, fear, separation anxieties and guilt on the part of family members. And as a behavior analyst, implement behavior programs to assist the resident in maintaining their skill level and improve their inappropriate behavior. As an active participant in the residents habilitation, the activity specialist can support, strengthen, and compliment other professionals involved in the treatment process insuring a team approach and continuity of care.

In summary, therapeutic activities are now an accepted mode of treatment being prescribed in facilities providing special care for residents suffering from Alzheimer's disease. Therapeutic activities, like all health services, have a specific purpose...to promote health, prevent increased disability, treat impairment and provide habilitation. For the activity specialist this is accomplished by developing, writing and implementing therapeutic activity program plans based upon the individual needs of the resident following a comprehensive assessment. And the one element which determines whether the activity is therapeutic or not is the method used in providing the service.

Therapeutic activities differ from the traditional recreational and leisure-time programs previously found in long-term care facilities. For example, therapeutic activities are written in a precise, specific and sharply defined manner and are goal directed. On the other hand recreational and leisure-time activities are just the opposite...they are general in nature, are not specifically written, are not goal directed and have little if any therapeutic value.

In conclusion, for an activity plan to be therapeutic it must contain four basic parts. They are:

1) Goals: Goals are vague, and subjective in nature. A goal defines the general direction in which the residents treatment plan will go. Goals are always written in a general but positive manner.

2) Objectives: Objectives are specific in nature and are goal directed. Objectives define the behavior desired when the resident completes his or her training. Objectives are always written in a very specific and positive manner.

3) Strategy: Strategies state the procedures that will be employed to assist the resident learn desired behavior or maintain skills levels. Strategies tell who will do the training, when it will be done, and how it will be done.

4) Evaluation: Evaluation is a means of monitoring a residents progress while he or she participates in training. These data collected will reflect whether the training is being successful, or not, and/or if the training is producing the desired results in his or her behavior that the objectives specify.

And finally, a therapeutic activity reflects a new and positive focus in working with residents suffering from Alzheimer's dementia. It places emphasis on the positive aspect of the residents behavior rather than on his or her problems. It places emphasis on what the resident can do for him or herself. It guards against putting a label on the resident and instead focuses on his or her behavior.

CHAPTER ONE

THE NURSING HOME. IT'S RESIDENTS AND THEIR PSYCHOLOGICAL PROBLEMS

If nursing home care is viewed realistically, the placement of individuals from the geriatric population in a nursing home facility does create problems for the resident. Although there are many problems which are at the same time being solved, placement in a nursing home precipitates a problem-loaded relationship between the home, resident, immediate family members, and close relatives, alike.

First of all, the resident resents the home because he or she is dependent, following a varying life span of productive independence. The end of his or her independence may be temporary, while on the other hand, it can very well be permanent. In essence, the resident gives up, or has taken away from him or her at the time of admission, many of the privileges he or she had previously enjoyed including the right to make decisions regarding his or her own life. All of a sudden, decisions are being made for him or her and he or she is in constant fear that the decisions may be wrong or may further take away what remains of his or her individuality. Since we are endowed with feelings of independence, it is natural for us as individuals to revolt against any unreasonable repression of it. And, acceptance of it can only come about through

1

traumatic episodes of regression. However, on one hand, some regression is desirable as it allows for acceptance of institutional therapy. On the other hand, it is undesirable because it must be overcome in order for rehabilitation to take place, and unless regression is complete, the revolt and rebellion against dependence will manifest itself in episodes of acting out, especially when family or friendly allies are present. And this rebellion, regardless of how subtle or passive, is generally disturbing to the individual who is visiting the resident in a home.

So, one major problem facing all residents in a nursing home facility is regression, the return to the state of a child-like dependency. It tends to be more severe during long periods of nursing home care. And, it is often associated with varying degrees of chronic brain syndromes due to the changes, malfunction and/or death of nerve cells of the brain, the latter taking form of symptoms commonly known as Alzheimer's disease which results in Dementia. And this combination of regression and senility results in a situation very similar to a child-like dependency and reactions which are rather morbid to any type of stimuli.

The stimuli, however, are perhaps most apparent during visits of a family member, close friend or relative. In far too many instances, the individual who is making the visit finds his visits unsatisfactory, and in many situations, right or wrong, cause him or her a great deal of stress. The underlying factor contributing to this is that the resident will usually seize upon this opportunity to express his or her dissatisfactions, whether they are real or imaginary, in an effort to get attention and attract some degree of sympathy.

The dependent situation in which the resident finds him or herself and his or her mixed feelings toward the home usually prohibits a direct and personal attack on nursing home personnel who serve him or her, except in unusual circumstances. And then it is likely to be somewhat passive and subtle. This is true largely because he or she fears retaliation or abandonment by the nurses and various other support personnel on whom he or she is dependent. Although he or she may be angry, rebellious, and lash out at nursing home personnel during the early stages of confinement, he or she will usually abandon this method. He or she will reject this rather unproductive means of fighting back because he or she knows the staff represents authority as well as being in the position of meeting and fulfilling his or her needs. And the frustration of having an enemy which he or she cannot attack directly results in his or her finding a solution to his or her problem by using family members or relatives on which he or she can project his or her hostility. The usual techniques are generally overt complaints or accusations of abuse and mistreatment which disturbs the family and creates a problem orientated situation.

The most trying and difficult reaction for the home as well as the family to handle is for the resident to completely reject the environment of the nursing home facility, his or her family, and any attempt to deal constructively with him or her. In such a situation, feelings of guilt are usually intensified. There is an underlying fear on the part of family members that the shock of separation from the family caused such a reaction in the patient. Many times this results in an unusual amount of anxiety on the part of the family involving the home's alleged inability to provide adequate care as well as environment.

In other situations, the resident will convey to the home and family, alike, that he or she is, in effect, too happy in his or her new surroundings. And their reaction, in return, seems to be that the nursing home through its efforts has made the resident so happy and content that he or she has no further need for family members, relatives or friends. This is, of course, in many instances, interpreted as rejection by the resident for family members. The family interprets his or her pleasure as a reflection of failure on their part to provide adequate care for him. And in such situations, the family may probe, explore, and question nursing home personnel in order to find something in the care or treatment which they can interpret as being neglectful or inadequate to use as an excuse for attacking the home. Of course, such an unreasonable attitude toward the home and its administration, although it may appear quite rational on the surface, should be explored in depth, understood and dealt with in an adequate and mature manner by nursing home personnel, family members and relatives alike.

It is at this point that the interdisciplinary team can come together and begin applying it's dissimilar professional skills and expertise to bare on defining and dealing with the residents maladaptive symptoms and/or behavior. It is during the admissions process that team members can begin to define many if not all of the residents psychological problems. In reality, the staff already knows a great deal about the resident prior to his or her admission based on their past experiences and accumulated knowledge about the trauma exhibited by the resident and his or her family prior to the admissions process. The staff knows, for example, that the resident experiences feelings of loss upon their admission to the nursing home facility. Loss of their independence, loss of control, loss of their dignity, loss of self-esteem, and self-worth which if not dealt with can lead to a major depression, separation anxieties or adjustment problems.

The team functioning in a preventive mode can through early detection, and intervention begin to define, target, and treat the residents mental, emotional and behavior disorders, and avoid a more serious episode of a mental disorder later during their tenure at the facility.

There are three categories of symptoms which the staff should look for when the resident is being screened for admission to their facility. The first category is the resident's feelings. The staff should monitor:

1) Feelings of anxiety, nervousness, worry and fear.

2) A feeling of losing control, thinks things around him or her are strange.

3) Feelings of being detached from all or part of their mental, emotional, spiritual, and physical being.

4) A feeling of apprehension, sudden and unexpected panic spells, and a sense of impending doom.

5) Feeling the tenseness, stress, and nervousness.

The second category of symptoms which the resident is likely to exhibit is their thought process. These symptoms are:

1) A difficulty in concentrating, jumping from one train of thought to another, and daydreaming.

2) Fears of losing control, of going crazy, fainting or passing out.

3) A fear of having a heart attack, death and of dying.

4) Fears of being left alone, of being deserted, isolated or abandoned.

5) A fear that something terrible is going to happen.

The third category consists of various physical symptoms or complaints by the resident.

The staff should monitor signs of:

1) A nervous and upset stomach.

2) Constipation or diarrhea.

3) A feeling of dizziness and lightheadedness.

4) Feelings of exhaustion or of being tired or run down.

Then, too, the resident might also exhibit a variety of symptoms which suggests possible depression which should alert the staff. They are:

1) Feelings of sadness – of being down in the dumps, or having the blues.

2) A feeling of being discouraged and helpless.

3) Feelings of low self – esteem, worthlessness, and failure.

4) A feeling of inferiority, and inadequacy.

5) Feelings of guilt, critical judgment of and blaming him or herself.

6) A feeling of irritability, frustration, resentfulness, and anger turned inward towards him or her self.

7) Feelings of a loss of interest in life.

8) A loss of motivation in everyday activities.

9) A poor self – image of being old and unattractive.

10) Poor appetite.

11) Reduction in social activity.

13) Chronic complaints about health.

14) Thoughts about death and dying.

Therapeutic activities can augment, support, strengthen, and compliment the services being provided by other professional disciplines on the team and contributes much to the treatment of the resident. For example:

1) Anything and everything you have learned in recreation, activities, or in life that promotes the strengthening, the flexibility and endurance of the resident's body and cognitive skills will invariably support your efforts to provide healing and promote well – being in the resident should be considered and implemented.

2) Exercise such as aerobic, swimming or walking can be productive.

3) Physical activities – such as yoga, stretching, dancing are all good ways to loosen the body and relieve stress and anxiety.

4) Massage to relieve stress, anxiety and tension.

5) For depression nurture the resident by taking walks in nature, viewing art, listening to good soft music, watching appropriate movies, television programs and gardening.

6) Experiment with different postures, i.e. head up, shoulders back and deep breathing exercises. All make the resident feel better. Try different ways of walking to see if some make the resident feel better than others.

7) Use meditation. A time for the resident to spend with him or her self.

8) Implement programs of viewing funny movies and papers, cassettes, funny books, cartoons, etc. to assist the resident with his or her anxiety and episodes of depression.

9) Schedule music sessions. Music does more than just soothe. It can stimulate or enhance almost any activity, emotion or mood.

10) Implement playful creative activities. Paint, write, sew, dance, cook, garden, sing, act, compose, play a musical instrument, a game, or sport.

11) Use education (both audio and video) to teach new skills for living a more productive satisfying and happy loving lifestyle.

The aim of prescribing therapeutic activities is to create a psychologically effective sequence of activities for those residents who exhibit symptoms or who are hurting because of a mental or emotional problem(s) upon entry into a nursing home environment. Often the activity director and/or specialist must design his or her own activity or modify an existing one to meet the resident's need(s). Therefore, it is essential for the activity therapist to be able to assess which features of an activity are likely to result in what behavior. Different activities require different behavior patterns from the residents. Therefore, when selecting or creating activities to achieve a treatment objective one must examine the terminal behavior desired and ask the question – Does the activity demonstrate the terminal behavior desired? If so, then implement the activity.

CHAPTER TWO

THE BEHAVIORAL APPROACH AND THERAPEUTIC ACTIVITIES

Advances in the field of mental health have led to the development of techniques and theories regarding the modification of human behavior. These techniques were developed primarily by experimental psychologists in their animal laboratories. And from the laboratories, the experiments gradually found their way into the helping professions including therapeutic activities in general where they have become known as behavioral theories and are behavior modification techniques. The basic underlying assumption of behavior modification is that behavior is not or does not occur at random, but, instead is lawful and as a result, is subject to prediction and control.

Thus, behavior modification can be productive when applied to the nursing home resident suffering from Alzheimer's disease. However, there are two primary difficulties which have been encountered in using behavioral modification techniques with residents of nursing homes: (1) There is a tendency for personnel applying it to focus too much of their attention on the undesired behavior and not to specify the behavior they want to see in the resident; and, (2) to develop a habit of turning to punishment in an attempt to eliminate the undesired behavior.

When applying behavior modification techniques, the first necessary condition is that personnel applying it specify exactly the type of behavior they want the resident to perform. It is not significant for personnel to say they want the resident to be good. Personnel must specify exactly what "good" means in terms of behavior and under what conditions, and exactly what criteria constitute being good. The expected behavior should be stated in a firm and positive manner. Personnel must specify exactly what the resident is expected to do. In reality, it is extremely difficult, if not almost impossible, to reinforce a resident for not doing something.

If personnel applying behavioral modification techniques do not specify exactly the behavior the resident should exhibit, then it is unreasonable to expect the resident to figure it out for him or herself. The first thing personnel must do is to be specific as to the behavior that is expected of the resident. And once the behavior has been clearly and specifically identified, the next step is to proceed in breaking down the terminal behavior and decide on the behavioral steps which can be implemented for the resident to go through to achieve the desired behavior. To expect the resident to know what behavior is expected of him or her is unrealistic. It is even more unrealistic to expect the resident to perform the desired behavior in a perfect manner before reinforcement is given.

It is possible, having set up these rules, to then specify a set of rules for the use of behavior modification techniques. The rules are as follows:

(1) The reward. Reinforcement should always follow the behavior immediately. This simply means that the amount of time elapsed between the occurrence of the task and the occurrence of reinforcing events should be near zero.

(2) The initial contact should call for small approximations. That is any small approximation of the desired response should be reinforced.

(3) All rewards should be given frequently in small amounts. This is important because frequent rewards are more likely to maintain the performance of the resident at a high level. And small reinforcements insure that the resident will not become saturated.

(4) The contract entered into between nursing home personnel and the resident must call for accomplishments rather than obedience. The resident who is reinforced for obedience rather than accomplishments is likely to become dependent on the individual attempting to implement behavior modification techniques in both his or her behavior and decisions. In essence, reinforcements for accomplishments is more likely to produce a resident who will be responsible for and able to control his or her own behavior.

(5) It is a must for all reinforcements to be presented immediately after the performance occurs. The procedure should first be performance, and then, reinforcement in that order because no resident learns on credit.

(6) It is important that the contract always be fair. Both the resident and nursing home personnel implementing the behavioral modification techniques must agree on the contract and its fairness. One should remember that it is not how the resident should see these situations, but, instead, how he or she actually sees it that really counts when attempts are being made to modify his or her behavior.

(7) And it is equally important that the contract be unanimously clear. The contract should be such that the terms are specifically stated.

(8) In addition to being clear, the contract must always be honest. A contract which is honest is one which is carried out according to the terms spelled out in the contract.

(9) It is of the utmost importance that the contract be a positive one. A workable formula for a contract is "I will do "X" if you will do "Y".

(10) It is also important to keep in mind that contracting must be used systematically. Personnel implementing behavioral modification techniques must continually remind themselves that the resident will cheerfully engage him or herself in an activity only if he or she knows that there is going to

be a payoff or reward. This is true because inconsistent use of positive reinforcement may lead to reinforcing undesirable acts on the part of the resident.

It has been found that individuals who apply behavioral techniques seem to exhibit a variety of biases. These biases seem to stem from their inner feelings and actions with residents. This is not good because these biases tend to undermine and work against the worker applying behavioral modification techniques in the sense that they usually prevent personnel from seeing the true interaction between themselves and the resident. In an effort to minimize this, personnel should focus on the behavior patterns which are undesirable. It is not unusual for personnel applying behavioral techniques to be able to specify very clearly exactly what it is that they do not like about a resident. They can describe the resident's behavior which they do not like and can usually specify the residents who exhibit the behavior more clearly. Furthermore, personnel applying behavioral techniques tend to ignore any good behavior that may be exhibited by a resident especially those who have been labeled as being bad.

Also, personnel tend to place far too much emphasis on punitive measures. In many instances, personnel are a lot more creative in methods of punishment than they are in methods of reward or reinforcement. They may go through an entire day administering a minimum number of rewards while at the same time spend a good portion of the day dispensing a variety of punishments as methods of controlling a residents behavior.

They also fail to specify desired behavior. Many individuals applying behavioral techniques are aware of the behavior they would like the resident to exhibit. They are far more conversant in what they do not want the resident to do rather than in what the desired behavior should be.

There is also a tendency on the part of personnel applying behavior techniques to dispense rewards or reinforcements independently of the residents behavior. It is not unusual for residents to be aware whether an individual is having a good or bad day or not with "good" or "bad" being designed as the tendency of the individual to pass out rewards such as a smile, a kind word, or a friendly pat on the back. If receiving a reward or reinforcement does not depend upon the residents behavior, but rather on something external to it, then the resident is deprived of the feed-back necessary for him or her to learn to respond to and at the same time, may well be on the way of learning behavior patterns that the same person applying the technique would later refer to as being inappropriate. Also, personnel who does not know the type of behavior they want the resident to exhibit and is aware of the role of positive reinforcement may still fail in their attempt to teach the resident because they expect too much too quickly.

Then too, personnel applying behavior modification techniques may have a tendency to label a resident as a result of generalizing from a few specific behavior patterns. One often finds the same individual responding to the labels they have provided and not to the resident. For example, a resident who acts in an anti-social manner may be labeled as "bad". From the point this label is applied, the resident will be treated as though he or she is bad regardless of any changes which he or she might make. While on the other hand, a "good" label may always be treated with favor even though the resident starts to exhibit inappropriate behavior. In any case, personnel applying behavioral techniques has ceased to respond to the resident and responds instead to a label.

One often finds that an individual's life has a bearing with the resident to the extent that their understanding of a resident communication is distorted. For example, a resident who says, "Mr. Doe, I don't like you" may really be saying "I don't like the nursing home" as readily as he is saying "I don't like the nursing home personnel". In either case, personnel applying behavioral techniques is taking the behavior of the resident exhibited personally without realizing that to many residents, nursing home personnel represents nothing more than part of a large system. When this misunderstanding has occurred, personnel applying behavioral techniques is likely to become de-sensitized and over-reactive to his or her further interactions with the resident.

In summary, behavioral therapy and/or counseling are terms frequently used in the same sense as behavior modification. All are derived from a conditional program. The Activity Specialist applying behavioral techniques should not view diagnosis and assessment traditionally as analytical descriptive activities, which specify what is wrong and sometimes what remedial measures should be taken. Instead activity personnel should begin with assumptions as to the nature of the psychological processes presumed to underlie the behavior problem. The problem is assumed to have developed as any other class of behavior through the natural operation of the laws of conditioning and learning. Behavioral problems can best be identified, analyzed behaviorally and distinguished by utilizing systematic and environment procedures to alter or shape a residents response to stimuli.

The activity staff applying behavioral techniques in their therapeutic activity programs should first make knowledgeable guesses about what reinforces and maintains undesirable behavior. And then he or she sets out to alter these in order to eradicate the behavior, produce a competing response, shape and mold appropriate behavior in the nursing home resident who is suffering from dementia.

CHAPTER THREE

EXAMPLES OF BEHAVIORAL OBJECTIVES TOPICS TO TEACH/ELIMINATE

Developing a global baseline checklist from which activity personnel can develop and implement goals and specific behavioral objectives for the nursing home population is not only desirable but necessary. However, developing such a comprehensive list of behavioral topics can be a challenge to some and aggravating to most activity therapists charged with implementing a therapeutic activity program in a nursing home facility. This task, however, can be made less complicated if the procedure is broken down into four broad categories. They are: 1) domiciliary, 2) social, 3) recreational, and 4) vocational. Since these four categories represent the normalization principal of the human species, specific behavioral objectives can be defined which represent all the behaviors the population residing in long term care facilities will need to make a satisfactory adjustment to the environment of a nursing home facility. In addition to topics which address the elimination of bizarre and/or disruptive behavior, they teach 1) self-help, 2) language, 3) social, 4) recreational, 5) academic and 6) vocational skills.

The following is a list of behavioral topics which can be considered or targeted for teaching or for eliminating inappropriate behavior in long term care facilities. The topics listed are those which are generally accepted as necessary for successful adaptation to the society in which we live with deficits severe enough in these areas to result in an individual to be labeled as being demented or deviant.

SELF-HELP SKILLS (TO TEACH)

Utensil feeding

Drinking from a cup

Drinking from a Glass

Table Manners

Toileting

Undressing

Dressing

Bathing

Showering

Tooth brushing

Hand and Face Washing

Shampooing

Hair Styling

Nail Care

Shaving – Face

Shaving – Arms and Legs

Menstrual Hygiene

Deodorant

Setting a Table

Make – Up

Food Preparation

Selects Clothes that Fit

Appropriate Style Clothes

Match Garments

Shoe Care

Clean and Mend Clothes

Press Clothes

Washer Operation

Dryer Operation

Crossing Sidewalks/ Intersections

Shopping

Cleaning House

Bed Making

Hanging Up Clothes

Fire and Safety

Personal First Aid

Traffic Lights

Sidewalks

Avoiding Moving Vehicles

Reading Signs

SOCIAL – ACTIVITY SKILLS (TO TEACH)

Gives Eye Contact to Familiar Persons

Watches Game as he Plays

Smiles/Laughs Appropriately

Gives Eye Contact to Strangers

Watches Game as Partners Play

Engages in Conversation

Makes Appropriate Comments

Normal Voice Inflection

Initiates Game

Not Too Aggressive

Does not Interfere With Others During Game

Games Have Reinforcement Value

Plays Games With Supervision

Cries appropriately

Normal reaction to strangers

Expresses Excitement Appropriately

Accepts Affection

Aware He Won the Game

Engages in Small Talk

Asks Questions

Shows Sympathy

Liked By Others

Apologizes When Appropriate

Friendly

Personal Appearance – Dress Right – Be Neat/Clean

Message the Resident Gives About Himself (Honest)

Break Time

Lunch Breaks

Dialogue with Staff

Punctuality

Smiles During Conversation

Normal Facial Expression

Not Too Shy

Takes Turns

Plays Normal Number of Games
(36 – 48)

Completes a Game

Plays Games Without Supervision

Differentiates Friends from Strangers

Expresses Anger Appropriately

Normal Display of Affection

Aware He Lost the Game

Appropriately Competitive

Initiates Small Talk

Answers Questions

Has a Special Friend

Patient

Polite

Enjoys People

Dialogue – Answering/Asking Questions

Maintains Good Posture

Bathroom

Dialogue with Peers

Health and Physical Condition

Absenteeism

SPECIFIC EXAMPLES OF BEHAVIORAL OBJECTIVES

TOILETING SKILLS (TO TEACH)

Goes to Toilet Alone, Defecates	Goes to Toilet Alone & Urinates
Trip Trained for Defecation	Trip Trained for Urination
Wipes With Tissue	Flushes Toilet
Washes/Dries After Toileting	Signals Staff Need To Leave Bed/Defecate
Signals Staff Need to Leave Bed/Urinate	Signals Staff Going to Urinate/Defecate
Places Self on Toilet	Places Self on Bedpan
Signals Staff in Need of Wiping	Bends Over, Raises Self When Wiped
Signals Staff When Ready to be Removed/Toilet	Signals When Ready to be Removed/Bedpan
Helps Staff Remove Self From Toilet	Helps Staff Remove Self From Bedpan
Signals When Ready To Be Removed from Toilet Area	

GROOMING SKILLS (TO TEACH)

Places Toothpaste on Toothbrush	Brushes Teeth With Toothbrush/Toothpaste
Uses Mouthwash	Washes Hair With Shampoo
Styles Hair	Dries Hair
Brushes/Combs Hair	Styles Hair to Normal Standards
Uses Hair Care Products Appropriately	Washes Hands at Sink
Dries Hands	Washes Face at Sink
Dries Wet Face	Bathes/Showers Self
Dries Body After Bathing	Trims and Cleans Nails
Mouth/Body Odor Acceptable	Applies Underarm Deodorant
Cleans Face	Blows Nose with Handkerchief/Tissue

Shaves Body Parts Appropriately

Applies Cosmetics Appropriately

Uses Skin Care Products Appropriately

Care for Personal Hygiene Needs

Wears Clothing That Fits Well

Wears Clothing of Approp. Style

Changes Clothing When Dirty

Changes Clothing When Torn

Wears Neatly Pressed Clothing

Matches Color Combinations

Wears Approp. Clothing/ Different Occasions

Wears Approp. Clothing/ Weather Conditions

Shine Shoes

Keep Shoes Clean

Keep Shoe Soles/Heels Repaired

Puts in Dentures/Plates

Keeps Clothing Free of Unusual Items

Cooperates When Being Groomed

Assists Staff When Placed in Tub/Shower

Washes Self in Tub/Shower

DRESSING SKILLS (TO TEACH)

Zips Zippers

Unzips Zippers

Snaps Snaps

Unsnaps Snaps

Button Buttons

Unbuttons Buttons

Ties Laces

Unties Laces

Hooks Bra (Female)

Unhooks Bra (Female)

Fastens Pants

Unfastens Pants

Buckles Buckles

Unbuckles Buckles

Puts On Underpants

Takes Off Underpants

Puts On Tee Shirt

Takes Off Tee Shirt

Puts On Bra (Female)

Takes Off Bra (Female)

Puts On Pants (Male & Female)

Takes Off Pants (Male & Female)

Put on Buttoned Shirt/Blouse

Takes Off Buttoned Shirt/ Blouse

Puts On Slip (Female)

Takes Off Slip (Female)

Puts On Dress (Female)

Takes Off Dress (Female)

Puts On Skirt (Female)

Takes Off Skirt (Female)

Puts On Socks

Takes Off Socks

Puts On Shoes	Takes Off Shoes
Puts On Coat	Takes Off Coat
Puts On Belt	Takes Off Belt
Puts On Suspenders	Takes Off Suspenders
Puts On Girdle (Female)	Takes Off Girdle (Female)
Puts On Panty Hose	Takes Off Panty Hose
Puts On Tie (Male)	Takes Off Tie (Male)

DINING SKILLS (TO TEACH)

Eats With Spoon Independently	Eats With Fork Independently
Eats With Knife Independently	Dining Room Independently
Eats From Plate Independently	Drinks From Cup/Glass
Walks To Table	Seats Self At Table
Sits Correctly At Table	Exhibits Approp. Table Manners
Drinks From Glass Without Spillage	Drinks From Cup Without Spillage
Drinks From Glass/Cup Silently	Approp. Utensils / Different Foods
Sucks Liquid From Straw	Plays With Food
Eats Too Fast	Eats Too Slow
Mouth Too Full	Spits Out Food
Eats Food From Table/Floor	Steals Food
Taps On Dish/Table With Utensils	Refuses To Eat
Eats Only Certain Foods	Talks With Food In Mouth
Swallows Liquids Appropriately	Finger Feeds
Uses Napkin While Eating	Uses Napkin To Wipe Mouth
Eats Finger Foods Appropriately	Eats Without Spilling Food
Keeps Mouth Closed While Chewing	Chews Food Before Swallowing
Asks Food To Be Passed	Serves Self From Bowl/Platter
Passes Bowl Without Spillage	Stands Up When Finished Eating
Pushes Chair Under Table	Leaves Dining Room Appropriately

PRACTICAL LIVING/ADL SKILLS (TO TEACH)
CLOTHES CARE

Hangs Clothing On Hanger	Takes Clothing Off Hanger
Folds Clothing For Storage	Puts Clothing In Proper Place
Folds Towels, Sheets, Etc.	Puts Towels/ Sheets in Proper Place
Separates Dirty Laundry	Identifies Laundry Supplies
Selects Appropriate Laundry Supplies	Measures Laundry Supplies
Washes Laundry By Hand	Uses Washing Machine
Uses Clothes Dryer/Clothes Line	Cleans Washer & Dryer
Cleans Lint Filter	Irons Clothing
Mend Tears	Utilizes Dry Cleaners/Laundry
Identifies Basic Sewing Equipment	Threads a Hand Needle
Sews on Buttons	Does Basic Hand Stitches
Pins & Cuts a Pattern	Operates a Sewing Machine
Selects Correct Dishes For Table	Sets Table
Clears Table After Meals	Cleans Off Dirty Dishes
Washes Dishes	Dries Dishes
Stores Dishes/Utensils Properly	Empties Garbage into Can Outside
Cleans Appliances	Clean/Straighten Kitchen Properly
Identifies Fruits	Identifies Vegetables
Identifies Dairy Products	Identifies Meats
Identifies Bread/Cereals	Identifies Foods Eaten Raw
Identifies Food Eaten Cooked	Select Food For Balanced Meal
Identifies Kitchen Equipment	Identifies Kitchen Furnishings
Uses Kitchen Equipment	Uses Kitchen Furnishings
Stores Kitchen Equipment	Uses Measuring Cups/Spoons
Operate Burners on Electric Stove	Operate Burners on Gas Stove

Operates Oven of Range

Interprets Recipes

Prepares Beverages

Makes Sandwiches

Makes Salads

Makes Desserts

Cleans/Prepare Basic Foods

Fries Basic Foods

Boils Basic Foods

Bakes Basic Foods

Prepares Precooked Foods

Prepares Combination Dishes

Plans Breakfast Meal

Plans Lunch Meal

Plans Dinner Meal

Prepare Breakfast Meal

Prepare Lunch Meal

Prepare Dinner Meal

Store Foods Properly

Recognizes Spoiled Foods

Cooks Meal in Sanitary Manner

Performs Safety in Kitchen

Knows Importance of a
Balanced Meal

SHOPPING SKILLS (TO TEACH)

Exhibits Correct Shopping
Behavior

Locates/Identifies Items in Store

Interprets Shopping List

Purchase Needed Items in Store

Ability to Shop Several Stores
During One Trip

HOUSEKEEPING (TO TEACH)

Vacuum Rugs

Sweep Floors

Mop Floors

Dust Furniture

Washes Walls/Windows

Straightens Room

Cleans Toilet

Cleans Bathtub/Shower/Sink

Changes Bath Towels When
Dirty

Makes Bed

Changes Bed Linen When
Dirty

Recognizes Need for Yard Work

Uses Hand Tools For Yard
Work

Uses Power Tools For Yard
Work

Knows Basic Plumbing

Knows Basic Electricity

Knows Basic Heating

Recognizes/Use Cleaning
Agents

TRANSPORTATION (TO TEACH)

Ride Bicycle	Ride Motorcycle
Drives Car	Uses Public Transportation
Observes Safety Rules	Crosses Street At Traffic Light
Crosses Street Without Traffic Light	Uses Sidewalks When Available
Uses Shoulder of Pavement When Sidewalk Unavailable	Walks Facing Traffic
Goes About Neighborhood Independently	Goes to Diverse Locations Independently
Travels to Neighboring Locations Alone	Travels to Distant Locations Alone
Avoid Unsafe Locations	

PUBLIC FACILITIES (TO TEACH)

Exhibits Correct Behavior at Public Events	Exhibits Correct Behavior in Restaurants
Exhibit Correct Behavior at Drive-In Restaurants	Exhibit Correct Behavior in Cafes
Orders Food Items At Fast Food Establishment	Orders Meals in Restaurants
Utilizes Vending Machines	Locates Public Restrooms
Use Public Restrooms	

PERSONAL INDEPENDENCE (TO TEACH)

Finds a Place To Live	Schedules Daily Routines
Uses Leisure Time/Activities Appropriately	Can Budget Time
Keeps Up With Personal Possessions	Maintains Proper Noise Level
Uses Ashtray/Matches Correctly When Smoking	Reports Fire/Evaluation Procedures
Avoids Environmental Hazards	Locks/Closes Windows and Doors

Locks and Unlocks Windows and Doors

Leaves Living Area Alone During Daytime

Leaves Living Area After Dark

Goes to Bed Unassisted

Mails a Letter Independently

Picks Up Mail Independently

Utilizes Post Office Facilities

Arranges For Utility Services

Locates And Acquires Medical Services

Locates Needed Social Services

Understands the Law

Cares for Minor Injuries/Burns

Recognizes When Hurt or Ill

SELF-ADMINISTRATION OF MEDICATION (TO TEACH)

Defines Kinds of Medication Taken

Identifies Med. By Size, Shape, etc.

Defines Amount of Medication to Take

Measures Liquid Medication

Reads Label on Medicine Container

Reads Numbers Letters on Syringe

Fills Syringe Properly

Gives Own Injection

Defines Time Medication is Ordered

Defines Consequences/ Medication Missed

Follows Instruction If Med Dosage Changed

Know How To Acquire Medication

Knows What to Do In Case of Reaction

Knows to Keep Med in Labeled Container

Knows When Medication May Be Omitted

Knows Not To Give Medication To Others

Administers Own Medication

Recognizes Unfavorable Reaction to Medication

Knows How To Use Non-Prescription Drugs

MOTOR COORDINATION (TO TEACH)

Walk with Normal Posture

Walk With Normal Gait

Begin to Show Hand Preference

Transfers Object Hand to Hand

Holds Object In Each Hand At Once

Turns Pages In Book, Singly

Scribbles With Pencil

Puts Rings Onto Stacker

Takes Rings Off Stacker

Puts Pegs Into Pegboard

Works Simple Puzzle

Touch Knee with Opposite Hand

Produces Freehand Drawing

Trace Pictures

Uses Paint Brush

Use Scissors

Copies Numbers

Prints Letters Independently

Prints Own Name

Prints Words Independently

Palmer Grasp

Reaches For an Object

Places Object in Large Container

Throw an Object

Catch an Object

Full Range of Neck

Full Range of Left Upper Extremity

Full Range of Left Lower Extremity

Functional Strength of Trunk Muscles

Functional Strength of Left Upper Extremities

Turn Head Side to Side – Supine Position

Support Self on Forearms in Prone Position

Takes Pegs Out of a Pegboard

Able to Complete Form board

String Beads

Touch Nose with Index Finger

Stencil Trace

Color Using Crayons

Paint with Water Colors

Copies Shapes

Copies Letters

Copies Words Independently

Writes Own Name

Write Cursive Script Independently

Pincer Grasp

Voluntarily Releases Object

Takes Object Out of Container

Kick an Object

Strike an Object with Hand

Full Range Right Upper Extremity

Full Range Right Lower Extremity

Functional Strength Neck Muscles

Functional Strength/Right Upper Extremity

Functional Strength of Left Lower Extremity

Lift Up Head/Upper Chest

Hold Head Even With Trunk of Body

Support Head and Chest on Extended Arms

Roll From Supine to Prone Position

Roll from Prone to Supine Position

Pull to Sitting Position from Lying

Hold Head Up & Steady when Sitting

Sit Alone With Good Balance

Move to & Maintain Hand-Knee Position

Move From Supine to Sitting Position

Pull to Stand Position

Stand Up From Sitting Position

Stand Independently

Good Posture While Standing

Walk Independently

Ascends Stairs with Aid

Ascends Stairs with Support

Ascends Stairs One Foot At a Time

Ascends Stairs Alternating Feet

Descends Stairs with Aid

Descends Stairs Using Handrail

Descends Stairs One Foot at a Time

Descends Stairs Alternating Feet

Jump From a Height

Jump Over an Object

Jump Onto an Object

Slide to the Left

Slide to the Right

Run

Acceptable Physical Endurance

Breathe Efficiently

Crawl

Creep on All Fours

Scoot in Sitting Position

Walks With Assistance of Another Person

Walks by Grasping Stationary Objects

Walks With Support of Walker, Crutches, Cane

Walks With Lower Extremity Braces

Walks Independently in Parallel Bars

Use of Wheelchair Independently

Sit in Wheelchair Without Support

Sit in Wheelchair With Support

Maneuver Wheelchair Without Assistance

Maneuver Wheelchair To Various Areas

Transfer From Wheelchair Independently

Transfer To Wheelchair Independently

Use Different Parts of
Wheelchair Appropriately

FOR BLIND ONLY

Ascend Stairs/Curbs With Sighted Guide	Descend Stairs/Curbs With Sighted Guide
Square Off With Sighted Guide	Go In/Out Door With Sighted Guide
Go Through Narrow Passages With Sighted Guide	Walk Along Sidewalk With Sighted Guide
Move Along a Wall Using Trailing Technique	Grip Cane Properly
Use Proper Cane Rhythm in Walking	Ascend Stairs/Curbs With Cane
Descend Stairs/Curbs With Cane	Go In and Out A Door With Cane
Go Through a Narrow Passage With Cane	Walk Sidewalk With Cane
React Properly to Traffic	Cross Street With Cane

EDUCATION (TO TEACH)
VISUAL DISCRIMINATION – COLORS, LETTERS, NUMBERS

Match Shapes	Match Colors
Match Letter Shapes	Match Single Digit Numerals
Match Double Digit Numerals	Match Simple Fractions
Identify Colors	Identify Primary Colors
Identify Secondary Colors	Names Colors
Names Colors of Objects	

IDENTIFICATION AWARENESS

Identifies Body Parts	Identifies Articles of Clothing
Identifies Pictures of Clothing	Identifies Animal Pictures
Identifies Furniture	Identifies Furniture Pictures
Identify Environmental Objects	Identify Environment Pictures
Names Articles of Clothing	Names Animals
Names Pieces of Furniture	Names Environment Objects

Names Pictures of Environment Objects	Names Body Parts

AWARENESS

Correctly Gives Part of Name	Correctly States Full Name
States Own Correct Age	Knows Own Gender
Name Place of Residence	States Correct Home Address, City
States Social Security Number	Identifies Self in Mirror or Photograph
Discriminates Dissimilar Sounds	Discriminates Similar Sounds
Recognizes Environmental Sounds	

NUMERICAL SKILLS

Count By Rote To Ten	Count By Rote To Twenty
Count By Rote To One Hundred	Count Objects To Ten
Count Objects To Twenty	Count Objects To One Hundred
Identify Single Digit Numerals	Identify Double Digit Numerals To Twenty
Identify Numerals To One Hundred	Print Numbers To Nine
Print Numbers To Twenty	Print Numbers To One Hundred
Count By Tens	Count By Fives
Adds Numbers Under Ten	Adds Double Digit Numerals
Adds Double Digits And Carries	Subtracts Numbers Under Ten
Subtracts Double Digit Numerals	Subtracts Double Digits and Borrow

IDENTIFICATION (PRE-READING)

Recite Letters Of The Alphabet	Print Letters Of The Alphabet
Recognizes Own Printed Name	

RECOGNITION OF BASIC TRAFFIC, SAFETY, WARNING AND DIRECTIVE SIGNS

Recognizes/Knows Meaning of Traffic Signs	Recognizes/Knows Informational Signs
Recognizes/Knows Meaning of Prohibitive Signs	Recognizes/Knows Meaning-Warning Signs
Able To Read Sight Words	Able to Read 2nd Grade Words
Able to Read 3rd Grade Words	Able to Read 4th Grade Words

TIME-TELLING SKILLS

Familiar With Concepts of Morning, Afternoon, Night	Recognizes Clock
Recognizes Long, Short Hands On Clock	Knows Function Of Clock
Tells Time of Daily Activities	Tells Time By Hour
Tells Time By The Half-Hour	Tells Times By The Quarter Hour
Tells Time By Fives	Tells Time By Minutes
Able to Set Clock	Able To Set Alarm Clock
Names Current Day of Week	Names Days of Week
Names Current Month of Year	Names Months of Year
Tells Current Date	Uses Calendar

TELEPHONE USE SKILLS

Knows Function Of Telephone	Dials a Phone Number
Place An Operator-Assisted Long Distance Call	Operate a Cell Phone
Call For Directory Assistance	Direct Dial A Long Distance Call
Use Telephone Directory Properly	Independently Use Telephone

Locate & Dial Emergency Numbers

Answers Telephone In Appropriate Manner

Takes/Writes Phone Messages

Follows Instructions Given Over Phone

Conveys Message To Others Over Telephone

MONEY MANAGEMENT SKILLS

Recognizes Money

Uses Money Appropriately

Identifies Penny, Nickel, Dime

Identifies Quarter, Half-Dollar

Familiar With Unitary Equivalency of Coins

Discriminates $1.00 and $5.00 Bill

Counts Money Combinations Up To $.25

Counts Money Combinations Up To $.50

Counts Money Combinations Up To $1.00

Counts Money Combinations $1/$5

Familiar With Unitary Equivalency Of Bills

Makes Change Up To A Quarter

Makes Change Up To a Half-Dollar

Makes Change Up To a Dollar

Makes Change Up To $5.00

Uses Mail To Pay Bills

Money Orders To Pay Bills

Utilizes Banking Services

Utilizes Checking Account

Budgets Money on Monthly Basis

SUPPLEMENTALS - LIBRARY

Holds Book Correctly

Looks Through Book Correctly

Chooses Library Book Without Assistance

Chooses Library Book With Assistance

Checks Out Library Book Without Assistance

Checks In Library Book Without Assistance

Uses Public Library With Assistance

Uses Public Library Independently

RECEPTIVE COMMUNICATION SKILLS (TO TEACH)

Speak in Complete Sentences

Use Pronouns, Adverbs and Verbs Tenses

Utilizes Sentences/Follows a Series of Commands

Responds to Questions

Utilizes Single Words/Follow Simple Commands

Responds To Sounds

Responds To Speech

Attends To Task

Obeys Simple Commands

Understands Concept of Commands

Identifies Common Nouns

Follows Simple Instructions

Follows One-Stage Command

Understands Difference In Objects/Pictures

Understands Common Verbs

Understands Prepositions

Follows Series of Simple But Related Commands

Understands Concepts Related to Shapes

Understands Concepts Related To Size

Understands Concepts of Temperature

Understands Concepts of Texture

Understands Concepts of Position

Understands Opposites

Categorizes According To Similarities

Formulates Judgment

Understands Past And Present

Understands Plural Nouns

Understands Plural Verbs

Comprehends Nouns-Verb Agreement

Understands Pronouns

Understands Future Tense

Understands Possessives

Understands Interrogatives

Understands Directions

Identifies Concepts Related To Height, Depth, Distance

Make Simple Decisions

Make Complex Decisions

Recognizes Common Labels

Attaches Label To Objects/ Pictures/Textures

Understands Sequential Order

HEARING IMPAIRED

Utilizes Visual Information

Communicates Using Auditory Cues

Speech Reading

Finger Spelling

Signing

Combines Signs & Finger Spelling

EXPRESSIVE COMMUNICATION SKILLS

Speech Is Easily Understood

Speech Is Intelligible

Speech Intelligible With Careful Listening

Speech Is Present/Limited

Vocalizations Present

Uses Non-Verbal Communication

Vocalizes Non-Speech Sounds

Vocalizes Speech Sounds

Uses Gestures

Imitates Sounds/Syllables

Produces Single Words

Express Needs By Gestures/ Vocalizations

Attempts New Words

Repeats Single Words

Uses Simple Phrases

Uses Declarative Sentences

Uses Interrogative Sentences

Uses Compound Sentences

Answers Questions

Uses Pronouns

Uses Possessives

Uses Plural Nouns

Uses Plural Verbs

Uses Adjectives

Uses Prepositions

Uses Conjunctions

Uses Adverbs

Defines Four Nouns

Expresses How Things Are Different

Expresses How Things Are Alike

Expresses Cause & Effect Of Relationships

Can Say Words

Retells Most Of Days Routine

Repeats Info. Sequential Order

Discusses Abstract Words Such As Love, Happy

Tells Occupations Of People

Describes Locations And Projects/Situations

Verbalizes Logical Choices/ Contingencies

Responses To Questions & Speech Appropriately

Normal Articulation

Has Mostly Intelligible Speech

Has Some Intelligible Speech

Normal Rate of Speech

Normal Volume of Speech

Normal Pitch of Speech

Normal Quality of Speech

PERCEPTUAL SKILLS

Visually Tracks An Object | Visually Attends To A Task

RECREATION SKILLS

Plays Games Appropriately
Plays Games With Supervision
Plays Games Without Supervision
Plays Structured Games Independently
Plays Unstructured Games Independently
Recognizes Winning Game
Recognizes Loss of Game
Shares Equipment With Others
Finds Peers With Whom To Play
Takes Turns Playing Games
Plays Games With Appropriate Equipment
Interferes With Progress During Activity
Plays With Bean Bag
Toss A Ball
Plays Simple Table Games
Plays Dominos
Plays Checkers
Plays Bingo
Plays Shuffleboard
Plays Card Games
Plays Basketball
Plays Catch
Plays Croquet
Plays Horseshoes
Plays Pool
Plays Putt-Putt Golf
Bowling
Cane Pole To Fish
Rod And Reel To Fish
Participates In Sporting Events
Attends Public Events
Attends Movie Theatres
Obtains Recreation Equipment/Supplies
Uses Public Media Schedules
Operate Television Set, CD Player/Radio

MUSIC

Moves Body Parts To Music
Moves In Rhythm To Music
Marches To Music
Complex Movements To Music
Selects A Rhythm Instrument
Plays Instrument To Music

36

Plays Instrument While Moving Body

Plays Rhythm Patterns

Sings

ART AND CERAMIC SKILLS

Moves Hands In Water

Uses Object In Water

Adjust Water Temperature

Cuts Objects From Paper

Uses Glue Properly

Works Clay With Hands

Assembles Clay Molds

Assembles Simple Molds

Assembles Complex Molds

Cleans Molds

Prepares Slip

Paints Ceramic

Prepares Green Ware

Creates Decorative Items

Select Appropriate Tools For Task

VOCATIONAL SKILLS

Punctual For Program

Follows Oral Directions

Waits For Directions Before Beginning Task

Completes Task In Allotted Time

Acceptable Stress Tolerance

Acceptable Work Tolerance

Adjusts To Job Change

Tolerates To Noise Level

Works With Supervision

Works With Minimal Supervision

Reacts Appropriately To Unusual Situations

Does Sedentary Work

Performs Light Work

Performs Medium Work

Performs Heavy Work

Has Appropriate Physical Stamina

Works Productively Alone

Interact Approp. With Co-Workers

Works Productively In Cooperative Work Setting

Works Productively In Parallel Work Setting

Works Productively In Close Proximity To Others

Socially Accepted By Co-Workers

Behavior Affects Productivity

Properly Maintains Work Station

Properly Cleans Work Area

Maintains Quality Standards Set/Employer

Uses/Stores Equipment Appropriately

Observes Safety Rules/ Procedures

Uses Time Clock Appropriately

Performs Duties of Cone Cleaner

Uses Counting Jig

Folds Materials To Given Size

Paints/Stamps Engineering Stakes

Pre-Measures Amounts of Material Needed

Weighs Items To Given Weight

Tears Materials To Approp. Sizes

Performs Simple Stocking Procedures

Performs as a Rag Sorter

Operates Drum Handler

Uses Commercial Hand Stapler

Counts Rapidly Up To Ten Items In Two Hours

Band Engineering Stakes

Discard Unwanted Items

Cut Material To Given Size

Discriminate Between Shapes, Colors/Sizes

Bundle Material

Use Manually Powered Equipment

Drive Small Nails, Tacks, Staples

Can Pull Tacks/Small Nails/ Staples

Mark Lines With Chalk

Thread Needles

Operate Sewing Machine

Remove Fabric From Furniture

Attach Fabric To Furniture

Prepare Fabric For Furniture

Identify Upholstery Equipment

Operate Button Machine

Prepare Foam For Use

Proper Use of Cleaning Supplies

Dust Work Area

Sweep Work Area

Mop Work Area

Wax in Work Area

Vacuum In Work Area

Buff In Work Area

Clean Windows

Clean Mirrors

Clean Ashtrays

Replenish Restroom Supplies In Work Area

Clean Waste Can

Clean Walls

Clean Bathrooms

Make And Change Beds

HORTICULTURE

Identify Tools For Soil Working

Identify Plants

Identify Basic Parts Of Plants

Use Tools For Soil Working

Prepare Soil For Planting

Plant Seeds

Plant Seedlings

Waters Plants Correctly

Identifies And Pulls Weeds

Identifies Ripe From Unripe Vegetables

Identifies Plants Needing Repotting

Identifies Potting Equipment/ Supplies

Identifies Potting Soil Ingredients

Mix Potting Soil

Cleans Dirty Pots

Pots A Plant

Knows Common Names Of Plants

Plants Shrubbery

Removes Shrubbery From Container

Plants Shrubbery In Hole

Fills Hole Around Shrub With Compost/Topsoil

Press Compost Around Shrubbery

Trench Soil Around Shrubbery

Mulch With Sawdust/Fine Straw

Select Appropriate Tools For Planting Shrubbery

Select Appropriate Tools For Planting Flowers

UNDESIRABLE BEHAVIOR (TO ELIMINATE)

No Eye Contact

Doesn't Look At Task

Doesn't Attend To Task

Uncooperative

Apathy

Temper Tantrums

Smears Feces

Short Attention Span

Hyperactivity

Gets Into Things

Eats Non-edibles

Rapid Change in Routine

Does Not Like To Be Interrupted

Won't Keep Clothes On

Runs Away

Bizarre Speech

Obscene Speech

Public Misbehavior

Over-dependent

Bad Table Manners

Nose Picking

Stopping Up Plumbing

Spitting

Destructive Behavior: Self/
Others

Hallucinations

Delusions

Hoarding

Wrong Sex Clothing

Ritualistic (Stereotyped)
Behavior

Panhandling

Exploitive Behavior

Repetitious Behavior

Screaming and Yelling

Drug And Alcohol Abuse

Stealing

Profanity

Echolalia

Negativism

Stealing Food At Meal Time

Does Not Like Affection From
Others

Inappropriate Sex

Inappropriate Touching/
Grabbing Others

Excessive Smiling

Bruxism

SPECIFIC MALADAPTIVE/DISRUPTIVE PROBLEM BEHAVIOR (TO ELIMINATE)

Self-Injurious: Head-Banging

Self-Injurious: Eye-Gouging

Self-Injurious: Swallows Foreign
Objects

Self-Injurious: Strikes Self

Self-Injurious: Bites Self

Self-Injurious: Cuts/Scratches
Self

Self-Injurious: Pulls Own Hair

Self-Injurious: Puts Into Body
Cavities

Self-Injurious: Pinches Self

Self-Injurious: Burns Self

Self-Injurious: Chokes Self

Physically Aggressive: Strikes
Others

Physically Aggressive: Cuts/
Scratch Others

Physically Aggressive: Pulls Hair

Physically Aggressive: Throws
Objects At Others

Physically Aggressive: Chokes
Others

Physically Aggressive: Bites Others

Physically Aggressive: Burns Others

Physically Aggressive: Sexually Assaults Others

Physically Aggressive: Pinches Others

Damages Property: Tears Own Clothing

Damages Property: Tears Others Clothing

Damages Property: Strikes Furniture

Damages Property: Throws Furniture

Damages Property: Breaks Windows

Damages Property: Sets Fires

Damages Property: Tears Curtains/Sheets

Damages Property: Vandalizes

Stereotyped Behavior: Body Rocking

Stereotyped Behavior: Hand Waving

Stereotyped Behavior: Head Weaving/Rolling

Stereotyped Behavior: Finger Waving

Stereotyped Behavior: Rubs Finger Tip & Thumb

Stereotyped Behavior: Staring

Stereotyped Behavior: Mimicking Others

Stereotyped Behavior: Rigid Posturing Limbs

Stereotyped Behavior: Rigid Posturing Body

Stereotyped Behavior: Arms Rigid

Stereotyped Behavior: Ritualistic Behavior Patterns

Stereotyped Behavior: Grinds Teeth

Inappropriate Sexual Behavior: Removes Clothing

Inappropriate Sexual Behavior: Exposes Body

Inappropriate Sexual Behavior: Public Masturbation

Inappropriate Sexual Behavior: Sexual Advances

Inappropriate Sexual Behavior: Promiscuity

Disruptive: Yells/Screams

Disruptive: Threatens Others

Disruptive: Spits On Others

Disruptive: Provokes Others

Disruptive: Night – Roams

Disruptive: Creates Disturbance/Night

Disruptive: Stops Up Toilet

Disruptive: Anti-compliant

Disruptive: Ignores Regs

Disruptive: Refuses To Follow Rules

Disruptive: Loud Behavior

Disruptive: Soils Self

Disruptive: Urinates on Self

Disruptive: Digs Feces

Disruptive: Plays W/Feces

Disruptive: Plays In Urine

Disruptive: Smears Feces

Disruptive: Throws Feces At Others

Disruptive: Steals Property

Disruptive: Uses Profanity

Disruptive: Hostile Language

Disruptive: Threatens Suicide

Bizarre Verbalization: Directed At Others

Bizarre Verbalization: Talks To Self

Bizarre Verbalization: Extreme Suspicions

Bizarre Verbalization: Persecution

Bizarre Verbalization: Repetition

Bizarre Verbalization: Abnormal Associations

Bizarre Verbalization: Irrelevant Content

Bizarre Verbalization: Visual Perceptions

Bizarre Verbalization: Distorted Reasoning

Bizarre Verbalization: Animal Sounds

Bizarre Verbalization: Mimicking Words

Problem Behavior: Begs Money

Problem Behavior: Hoards Objects

Problem Behavior: Inappropriate Noises in Public

Problem Behavior: Wears Unusual Objects

Problem Behavior: Stuffs Pockets With Objects

Problem Behavior: Excessive Use Of Drugs

Problem Behavior: Social Withdrawal

Problem Behavior: Ticks

Problem Behavior: Extreme Avoidance

Problem Behavior: Hyperactive Cycle

Problem Behavior: Seizure Activity

Problem Behavior: Result of Changes

CHAPTER FOUR

WRITING BEHAVIORAL GOALS

Goals are a vital part of any treatment plan. They define the general direction in which the treatment process will proceed. Also they motivate the activity specialist and interdisciplinary team members to focus on the specific needs of the resident – what he or she can do, needs to do and wants to do to improve or maintain their skill level and quality of life. Then too, it drives the activity specialist and team members to concentrate on and consider what they as caregivers need to do to motivate the resident to participate in the activity plan.

Goals are one of four basic parts of a treatment plan. However, writing goals requires thought, insight and prior observation into the residents behavior. And, to achieve such insight into his or her behavior, a comprehensive analysis of the residents behavior must be done as it defines the resident's strengths and needs. Such a comprehensive evaluation of the resident defining his or her strengths and needs serves to ensure a well – developed and scientifically documented approach to formulating and writing positive, technically sound, and measurable goals.

In addition to one's own assessment, evaluations from other professional disciplines are of significant value in developing the residents strengths and needs list from which the goals are derived. Also, every effort should be made to involve the resident because they are able to give valuable information which often contributes to the addition of data which might otherwise be overlooked or omitted which will compliment and enhance the strengths and needs list which will ensure well crafted goal statements. Then, too, input from immediate family members, relatives, support personnel and caretakers who provide direct hands – on care can be of significance in assisting the activity specialist and team members in defining and developing the residents goals.

Goals are essential in the process of developing a sound and meaningful plan of treatment. The foundation of any effective treatment plan relies on the data collected prior to the writing of the plan. Therefore, all data should be collected in a serious and respectful manner and done so by doing a thorough bio-psychosocial evaluation. As the resident and family members are interviewed the activity specialist and team members must listen sensitively. They must try to understand and process what the resident and family members are struggling with such as family issues, stressors, mental and emotional problems, support groups, physical health problems, coping skills, interpersonal relationships or lack of self – esteem, loss, separation and adjustment issues. When doing a comprehensive assessment the activity specialist should mesh and integrate not only the data obtained from the individual assessment but also from team members who have evaluated the resident. This is a critical step in understanding the resident, his or her family and the mental and emotional struggles in which they are trying to cope.

Goals should be formulated adhering to the team concept of team input and the process should begin by defining and developing a strengths and needs list. The resident's strengths list will assist the teams ability to define what the resident can do, would like to do, and is willing to do. And from the need's list the team will be able to define what the team wants the resident to do and what the resident would like to accomplish.

From the residents assessments the team must single out and prioritize the most significant problems on which to focus during the treatment process. And, with the elderly resident, especially those suffering from Alzheimer's Disease, with cognitive impairment, such problems may be singled out by a family member caregiver or other healthcare provider. Usually primary problem(s) of concern will surface and secondary problem(s) will follow. The reason they should be prioritized into Priority I and Priority II Goals primarily is to define immediate needs, requiring attention and to maintain a sense of direction and continuity during treatment.

As goals are being selected it should become clear to the team members how important it is to include opinions from all who have a vested interest in the resident and the importance of the goals which reflect the issues for the resident that requires help. The team should not ever forget that the residents motivation to participate in his or her treatment depends greatly on the degree in which the treatment process addresses their greatest needs.

Goals selected for treatment should focus on how a problem and/or need reveals itself behaviorally in a resident's life – how it affects his or her quality of life. Therefore, goals are defined and formulated for the resolution of, or to improve, reduce, or maintain targeted problem areas. These goals statements should be developed and written in measurable terms that indicate a desired positive outcome during the treatment process.

The elderly resident entering, or living in, a long-term care facility are not always capable, due to decreased cognitive skills, to decide for themselves what they want to do, nor are they always able to participate in devising their own systematic procedures for achievement. Therefore, the activity specialist and team members must assist in helping him or her define the goals which they need to pursue, which are desirable, achievable and controllable.

A helpful method to begin to define and develop the resident's strengths and needs list is to think positively about the resident instead of thinking about what he or she lacks. This should always be a consideration because when a resident's needs are met, he or she will develop more strengths.

The following is an example of how a strengths and needs list might be formulated from which goals are developed and prioritized:

> The nursing home facility which specializes in providing special care for Alzheimer's residents has just admitted Mr. Sam Sad, a 79 year old Caucasian male for services. As Director of the activity program at the facility you have reviewed his admission's history and know that Mr. Sad has been diagnosed by his attending physician and consulting psychiatrist as having dementia of the Alzheimer's type and appears to be in Stage Five (5) or Stage six (6) of the disease.
>
> By history, Mr. Sad was recently widowed after forty-five

(45) years of marriage. His wife died after a long and costly battle with cervical cancer. He is the father of three children and three grandchildren. Mr. Sad is a college graduate, and by profession was an accountant and C.P.A. He has been retired for several years and after retiring built and flew model aircraft as a hobby – he was a fighter pilot during World War II.

Mr. Sad was admitted three (3) days ago and a team meeting has been scheduled with activity personnel to develop and write an individual therapeutic activity plan for Mr. Sad. Mr. Sad was in attendance but was quite, had little to say, and sat staring into space with a fixed smile on his face. He seemed to be experiencing weight loss, was clean, neat and well groomed, however, his clothing was wrinkled, the fly of his pants was unzipped, and there was evidence of coffee and food stains on his shirt. He had a nice selection of clothing and from reports he always took pride in dressing appropriately, buying the latest style of clothing whether he needed them or not. However, he tended to, if he wasn't assisted, to wear the same clothing everyday or would wear articles of clothing that did not match. His speech, although good, was slow and blocking, at times. He often used inappropriate curse words, vulgarity, and expressions in an effort to make a point. He has good range of motion of his upper and lower extremities.

His posture was good, as was his gait and balance. His memory was poor especially his ability to recall current events. His state of awareness was poor – lost in time. He believed that he still had responsibilities especially towards his deceased wife, home, family, and job. He didn't believe he required assistance, his perception of reality was based upon misperceptions. And he retained some abilities to form thoughts, plan an action, and follow – through on them. Mr. Sad's behavior was generally poor in that he had good social skills during the morning hours but it deteriorated as the day progressed. He had a habit of wandering looking for an exit, attempting to elope and losing his sense of direction and train of thought. He was at times suspicious, kept to himself and had a lot of anxiety which seemed to be related to his short memory span which resulted in his misconceptions. He had bouts of crying and often seemed depressed.

Mr. Sad needed assistance with ADLs and gave a lot of resistance to caregivers with whom he was unfamiliar. His ADLs required some simplification and extension of time in dining, toileting, bathing, dressing, and grooming. He had a sleep disturbance, didn't interact well with others, had a fear of being left alone, had some pre-occupation with sexual activities and was having trouble being separated from his family and of adjusting to a nursing home environment.

Mr. Sad had been residing with his children. They took turns in caring for him. They decided on placing him in a long – term care facility because they could no longer maintain him in their home and community because of his inappropriate and unacceptable behavior, I.e.. inappropriate sexual comments and gestures toward women. His family was active in his habilitation.

After critiquing Mr. Sad's history, his strengths and needs might look like the following. Remember, the Strengths List should reflect what the resident can do, likes to do, and individuals who are willing to help. The Needs List should reflect what the team would like and need to accomplish.

STRENGTHS:	NEEDS:
1) Has excellent family support.	1) Reduce wandering.
2) Ambulation is very good.	2) Improve language skills.
3) Likes flying and model airplanes.	3) Improve social skills.
4) Alert during morning hours.	5) Improve toileting skills.
5) Enjoys selecting and wearing clothing.	6) Improve bathing skills.
6) Liked to have good selection of clothing.	7) Improve grooming skills.
7) Able to communicate his wants/needs.	8) Improve dressing skills.
8) Good usage of upper extremities.	9) Improve dining skills.

I) Guidelines for writing goals.

When writing goals they should be written in short simple, and everyday language. They should always be stated in a general and positive manner stating the direction in which training will proceed as indicated in the following examples.

1) Improve social skills.

2) Improve dining skills.

3) Improve dressing skills.

4) Improve bathing skills.

5) Improve grooming skills.

6) Improve toileting skills.

7) Reduce wandering.

8) Improve language skills.

9) Improve proper exercises.

II) Priortizing goals.

After the goals have been listed, they are prioritized into Priority I and II level goals. Priority I goals will be the goals the team members consider are the ones that the resident needs to work on immediately and in most situations are limited to no more than three (3) at a time. As Priority I goals are completed, Priority II goals will be moved up and become Priority I goals for the resident on which to work.

Examples of Priority I Goals.

1) Reduce episodes of wandering.

2) Teach appropriate social skills.

3) Teach appropriate language skills.

Examples of Priority II Goals.

4) Teach proper exercise skills.

5) Teach appropriate dining skills.

6) Teach appropriate grooming skills.

7) Teach appropriate bathing skills.

8) Teach appropriate toileting skills.

III) Goals should be relevant.

Goals should address those skills which will be beneficial or useful to the resident. There is little value in investing time and energy teaching the resident a skill or skills which he or she could just as well do without. The most relevant skills are those which the resident needs and will use to function in his or her environment – those practical living skills such as toileting, bathing, grooming, dressing, and dining. However, regardless of the skill or skills selected to be taught, the skills must be clearly specified and defined before goals can be written. Having precisely written goals are essential for successful completion. Goals must always be written based on the individual needs of each resident, and upon a diagnostic assessment. They must be measurable, have a start and completion date, reflect team input and continuity of care.

IV) When targeting goals are to be taught, limit them to two or three at a time.

From the strengths and needs list come far more goals than the staff and resident have the time or energy on which to work. The tendency to list too many goals is never an accepted practice because attempting to work on too many goals at any time is confusing. This is one of the reasons why goals, after they are listed, are prioritized into Priority I Goals and Priority II Goals. After deciding on what goals are going to be taught and effective teaching techniques are implemented the goals should be written in a simple manner, broken down into small steps and be both practical and relevant.

V) When listing goals consider the sequence of development.

When developing and prioritizing goals, one should take into account which goal or goals need immediate attention, keeping in mind that goals must always be limited to what seems practical at the time. There are instances when goals which are written are too ambitious for the resident. So a good rule to follow is to always make sure that they are stated in a simple manner and broken down into the smallest of steps possible. Also many skills and/or behaviors are learned in sequence. Therefore, rather than teaching a resident to eat with a spoon, it would be best to teach him or her how to first grasp eating utensils.

VI) Both short and long term goals should be considered.

It is important to consider both. Short term goals will permit the resident to make progress and keep him/her from becoming discouraged during the treatment process. Long term goals are necessary. They indicate what the treatment plan will eventually accomplish, however, long term goals can be difficult for the resident and in many situations take months and years to complete. Decisions about the practicality of a goal or goals should be based upon natural hierarchies. There are certain behavioral prerequisites which have to be taught, i.e. To teach a resident to fold a wash cloth must first be taught to attend to a task for more than a few seconds. In other words, one always begins with the basics and gradually builds up to a more elaborate and difficult task. By beginning with tasks which are the most essential to complete, other higher level tasks will become possible.

VII) It is important to be realistic.

Teaching goals must always be limited to what seems realistic at the time. Although long term goals may be ambitious immediate goals should be more modest. For example, a resident who paces the ward at night disturbing others would need a goal which addresses his or her hyperactivity. From his or her social history one of his or her needs is to improve his or her grooming program would not be realistic. Perhaps a more realistic and appropriate goal would be to teach him or her to sit quietly in a chair.

VIII) Goals should be important and meaningful.

The general statements of goals, although limited in usefulness because they don't always tell you exactly what you want the resident to do, permit staff to establish some general guidelines for treatment without requiring one to be too precise. Since goals are, by nature, vague and usually subjective and define the general direction of the resident's treatment plan, it is vital that the goals always be positive, understandable to the staff, important and meaningful to the resident.

A REVIEW OF WRITING GOALS.

I. Definition:

*Goals are VAGUE;

*They are usually SUBJECTIVE and GLOBAL in nature;

*They are written in a positive language to define the GENERAL DIRECTION in which the residents treatment plan will proceed.

II. The Ten Categories FROM which goals are generally derived are:

*Bizarre and Inappropriate Behavior;

*Motor Deficits;

*Self-help Skills;

*Practical Living Skills (ADLs);

*Language Skills;

*Social Skills;

*Recreational Skills;

*Academic Skills;

*Vocational Skills;

*Cognitive Skills.

III. Some examples of TOPICS and METHODS for writing goals:

*Improve Recreational Skills;

*Reduce Fears of Loss;

*Improve Interpersonal Relationships;

*Reduce Incidents of Non-participation in Activities;

*Improve Social Skills;

*Reduce Episodes of Anger;

*Improve Adjustment Skills;

*Teach Appropriate Gestures;

*Improve Physical Stamina;

*Reduce Fears of Desertion;

*Reduce Self Esteem;

*Identify Environmental Objects;

*Reduce Episodes of Withdrawal From Social Events;

*Teach Appropriate Language Skills;

*Reduce Separation Anxieties;

*Improve Greeting Skills;

*Reduce Fears of Death and Dying;

*Improve Self Worth;

*Increase Attention Span;

*Relate Positively To Others During Activities;

*Improve Housekeeping Habits;

*Develop Good Work Habits;

*Improve Self Confidence;

*Lift a ½ Lb. Weight;

*Teach Appropriate Manners;

*Teach Appropriate Social Graces.

CHAPTER FIVE

WRITING BEHAVIORAL OBJECTIVES

The purpose of writing objectives is to make it as clear as possible to staff members and residents alike what activity needs to be taught, when it is to be taught, who is going to teach it, where the training will take place and how it will be done. Objectives tell in specific behavioral terms what the team members want the resident to accomplish and be able to perform upon completion of the prescribed program.

The establishment of objectives is the heart and soul of any treatment plan. The aim of writing objectives is to develop psychologically effective sequences of an activity through which a specific objective on the part of the resident can be achieved and which will have maximum impact on his or her behavior.

Objectives are generally formulated and written in three areas: 1) cognitive (thinking), 2) motoric (doing), and 3)affective (feeling). These areas, however, are interrelated and focus on one primary targeted objective. However, any and all objectives must always be written in a specific manner and be measurable, observable, desirable, controllable, attainable, realistic, and time-sensitive. Objectives most always reflect the following:

1) Performance means actually doing something. The statement of performance must specify behavior that can be observed;

2) Conditions means that the objective must clearly state the conditions under which the performance is to take place, and;

3) Extent means that the behavioral objective must establish an acceptable minimal level of achievement.

When formulating and developing objectives the following principals must be included:

1) Specify terminal behavior – First identify the behavior and then determine how it is to be measured;

2) Baseline – Assess residents behavior to determine correct level of functional or non-functional behavior;

3) Structure a favorable situation – Provide resident the opportunity to exhibit appropriate behavior rather than just inappropriate behavior.

4) Establish motivation – Define appropriate re-enforcers and/or locate, withhold, deprive if necessary, re-enforcers, if and when the resident exhibits inappropriate behavior;

5) Adaptation – To extinguish emotional respondents, provide and/or establish discriminative stimuli, and establish reinforcer;

6) Shape desired behavior – Reinforce desired behavior, raise/reduce criteria for reinforcement gradually, present reinforcement immediately.

7) Keep continuous objective records.

As objectives are written, in addition to one's own assessment, evaluations from other professionals are of significant value in developing a strengths and needs list from which objectives are derived. Then, too, input from family members, relatives, caregivers and support personnel is also of great value in developing objectives of the resident.

In review, when writing objectives they are very specific and goal directed. Objectives are precise. They are broken down into several small simple steps. They tell the staff exactly what the resident will do, how he or she will do it, and when training is completed. Objectives move away from general statements of a program's intentions to a very specific definition of the skill and/or behavior the staff wants the resident to exhibit when the objective is completed.

An important first step to remember in writing objectives is to specifically define what the resident can and cannot do. Therefore, the first step in writing objectives is to obtain and record of the operant level of the behavior – exactly pinpointing the step and/or level at which the resident cannot perform a task and/or behavior. The staff must establish the level at which the behavior is occurring before he or she attempts to modify it. This record of the operant level of the behavior is called a baseline. A baseline, therefore, is a pre-experimental record of a behavior and tells the staff at what step the resident should begin training when working on an objective. Very briefly the procedure of base lining can be summarized as follows:

1) The behavior must be specifically and clearly defined;

2) Once the behavior is specifically defined, the operant or baseline level of the behavior is recorded. The level of the behavior must be measured as it is occurring before any attempts are made to change it;

3) Once the level at which the need or behavior is established, the training procedures are then instituted;

4) The recording of the behavior is then continued. This provides continuous feedback to the trainer as to the effectiveness of the training and indicates if further training procedures are necessary.

Once the baseline is completed and the level at which training will begin objectives are written. Remember objectives are written very specifically and are goal directed. Objectives serve a specific purpose. They are important in that they provide guidelines for both the staff and resident. Objectives explain in detailed terms exactly what the staff wants the resident to do. For example:

Example 1) Goal: John will drink from a glass, (or drink from a glass).

Objective: John will pick up his glass, raising it to his mouth with verbal prompts 3 times during each meal for 10 consecutive meals by _____.

Example 2) Goal: John will use a bath cloth, (or use a bath cloth).

Objective: John will tolerate a damp bath cloth to be rubbed on the side of face with hand over hand assistance 1 time during each shift for 10 consecutive shifts during his bath, by _____.

Example 3) Goal: John will use a towel, (or use a towel).

Objective: John will dry his face with a towel with gestural prompts 3 of 5 times each day on 8 consecutive days, by _____.

Example 4) Goal: John will exercise arm muscles, (or exercise arm muscles).

Objective: John will use his arm muscles with physical assistance by reaching for a towel on 3 of 5 occasions each day for 8 consecutive days, by _____.

Example 5) Goal: John will improve his social skills, (or improve social skills).

Objective: John will look at another person during small group therapy sessions with verbal prompts 3 of 5 times during a session for 10 consecutive sessions, by _____.

Example 6) Goal: John will exercise his leg muscles, (or exercise leg muscles).

Objective: By _____, John will walk 5 minutes each day independently, with physical prompts, on 3 of 5 trials without stopping for a rest on 5 consecutive days.

Example 7) Goal: John will do push-ups for exercise, (or do push-ups).

Objective: By _____, John will do 5 push-ups per 1 minutes 3 of 5 trials with gestural prompts on 5 consecutive days.

Example 8) Goal: John will swim to exercise chest muscles, (or exercise chest muscles).

Objective: By _____, John will swim for ½ hour every day, on 3 of 5 trials, with physical prompts on 5 consecutive days.

Example 9) Goal: John will make eye contact, (or make eye contact).

Objective: By _____, John will make eye contact when trainer calls his name at 20 minute intervals on 3 of 5 trials for 5 consecutive days.

Example 10) Goal: John will state time correctly, (or state time correctly).

Objective: By _____, John will state the time of day to the minute correctly with verbal prompts by trainer on 3 of 5 trials on 5 consecutive days.

Example 11) Goal: Walk for Exercise.

Objective: Within _____, John will walk to and from the dining room independently with verbal prompts on 3 of 5 trials on 5 consecutive days.

Example 12) Goal: Use wheelchair.

Objective: Within _____, John will use wheelchair to transport himself to and from the dining room without assistance with verbal prompts on 3 of 5 trials on 5 consecutive days.

Example 13) Goal: Obeys simple commands.

Objective: Within _____, John will carry out one stage commands with verbal prompts 4 of 5 times on 5 consecutive days.

Example 14) Goal: Repeat single words.

Objective: Within _____, John will repeat single
words intelligibly with verbal prompts on 4 of 5
trials on 5 consecutive days.

Example 15) Goal: Move to rhythm of music.

Objective: Within _____, John will move to rhythm
of music with verbal prompts on 4 of 5 trials on 3
consecutive days.

In these examples the goals state the general direction that the program will take, but does not indicate specifically what the residents behavior will be nor when he or she will complete the task. On the other hand, objectives are very specific. They: 1) describe the behavior that can be observed and measured. 2) are outcome orientated as it tells us what the residents behavior will be at the conclusion of training and 3) they are time-linked in that they specifically tell us how long it will take the resident to learn and/or master the task or behavior. Behavioral simply means, in the final analysis, that objectives specify behavior which are both observable and measurable.

The preceding examples show how goals and objectives are different and yet are also alike. For example, objectives are generally different from goals in that objectives describe observable, measurable, behavior, are outcome-orientated and are time linked. On the other hand, objectives are like goals in that they emphasize competency, and not deviancy, are written in positive language, reflect sequential and progressive behavior, are realistic, and they are understandable to the staff and the resident alike.

In conclusion, goals and objectives are the heart and soul of any treatment plan. And each plan must be individualized and tailored to the resident's particular problems and needs. Treatment Plans are never mass – produced, even if residents have similar needs, a resident's strengths and needs, unique stressors, support systems, family situations, behavioral patterns and symptoms must be assessed and critiqued in developing a treatment plan and strategies. Such an approach will promote an effective and creative treatment plan, which will not only benefit the resident but the Activity Specialist and team alike.

BARRIERS AND SOLUTIONS

Before a final decision is made about how and when an objective will be accomplished and which staff member(s) will do the training, it is wise to define possible "barriers" that might interfere with the resident(s) passing the objective(s) and possible solutions to eradicate these barriers. There are four basic and fundamental barriers, other than medical, which should always be examined before an objective is activated: 1) behavior problems, 2) unacceptable social behavior, 3) cultural deprivation and 4) limited cognitive skills.

Barriers might include needs for prerequisite training in one or all of the above listed fundamental barriers in which case the objective(s) might be revised or a new objective and strategy written to address this need(s). Also a barrier(s) could be problems with such things as transportation, scheduling, space for training, lack of personnel, or the need to solicit the cooperation of other individuals who will be involved in the training process. And the strengths and needs list is always an excellent source for identifying barriers as well as solutions.

EXAMPLE: Objectives are being written for John who was recently admitted for skilled nursing home care because he had been diagnosed as having Alzheimer's disease. In reviewing John's strengths and needs list it was noticed that John was taking psychotropic medication for depression which seemed to be interfering with his sleep cycles and energy level. The team felt this presented a barrier to his being able to participate in or complete on schedule the goals and objectives assigned to him in self-help and practical living skills. The team in an effort to find a solution decided to refer John to the local behavior health center for a psychiatric assessment to include a review of the psychotropic medication he was taking. In addition the team members also recommended that a behavior management plan be developed to augment the treatment being prescribed by the psychiatric staff at the behavior health care facility. John would not begin training until these proposed solutions were completed. Thus a barrier was defined and a solution(s) was developed to deal with it.

I. A Review of Writing Objectives.

Definition:

*Objectives tell in behavioral terms exactly what you want your resident to DO when he or she completes a particular segment of training;

*Objectives are SPECIFIC and GOAL DIRECTED;

*They are OUTCOME – ORIENTED;

*They are TIME – LINKED;

*They have a BEGINNING and COMPLETION DATE;

*They mandate that behavior can and must be OBSERVED, MEASURED, RECORDED and TRACKED;

*They tell HOW LONG;

*They tell HOW MUCH;

*They tell HOW OFTEN;

Example:

Goal: Ms. Doe will adhere to a schedule.

Objective: Within six (6) months (HOW LONG) (1 September 2004) Ms. Doe WILL state the time of day correctly (HOW MUCH) to the minute on eight (8) of ten (10) trials (HOW OFTEN) when verbally instructed to do so by trainer.

II. A Review of Some Examples of Goals and Objectives.

1) Goal: Improve/Maintain Social Skills:

Objective: Ms. Doe will relate positively to others during daily social events on Monday, Wednesday and Friday of each week when verbally prompted to do so by Trainer by 1 October 2004.

2) Goal: Improve/Maintain Participation in Activities:

Objective: Ms. Doe will improve her "physical stamina" by walking for fifteen (15) minutes without stopping for rest on every day of week when verbally prompted to do so by trainer by 1 October 2004.

3) Goal: Improve/Maintain Adjustment skills:

Objective: By 1 October 2004 Ms. Doe will relate positively to others and to nursing home environment on Monday, Wednesday and Friday of each week when verbally prompted to do so by trainer.

4) Goal: Reduce Separation Anxieties:

Objective: Ms. Doe will reduce her incidents of persistent verbalization and sematic complains about separation from family or attachment figures to five (5) episodes per day per week when physically prompted to do so by the trainer by 1 April 2004.

5) Goal: Become More Independent:

Objective: Within six (6) months (1 August 2004) Ms. Doe will board bus to participate in community awareness program by herself each day on time for the event when verbally prompted to do so by trainer.

Some Examples of Long Term/On-Going Goals and Objectives

Goal 1. Ms. Doe will improve her social skills.

Objective 1.1 Ms. Doe will relate positively to her peers and to significant others during social events on Monday, Wednesday, and Friday of each week when physically prompted to do so by Trainer by 1 April 2004.

Objective 1.2 Ms. Doe will relate positively to her peers and to significant others during social events on Monday, Wednesday, and Friday of each week when gesturally prompted to do so by Trainer by 1 July 2004.

Objective 1.3 Ms. Doe will relate positively to her peers and to significant others during social events on Monday, Wednesday and Friday of each week when verbally prompted to do so by Trainer by 1 October 2004.

Objective 1.4 Ms. Doe will relate positively to her peers and to significant others during social events on Monday, Wednesday, and Friday of each week independently by 1 January 2005.

Goal 2. Improve Participation in Activities.

Objective 2.1 Ms. Doe will improve her "physical stamina" by walking for three (3) minutes without stopping for rest on every day of week when verbally prompted to do so by the Trainer by 1 April 2004.

Objective 2.2 Ms. Doe will improve her "physical stamina" by walking for six (6) minutes without stopping for rest on every day of week when verbally prompted to do so by the Trailer by 1 July 2004.

Objective 2.3 Ms. Doe will improve her "physical stamina" by walking for nine (9) minutes without stopping for rest on every day of week when verbally prompted to do so by the Trainer by 1 October 2004.

Objective 2.4 Ms. Doe will improve her "physical stamina" by walking for twelve (12) minutes without stopping for rest on every day of week when verbally prompted to do so by the Trainer by 1 January 2005.

Goal 3: Improve Adjustment Skills.

Objective 3.1 By 1 April 2004 Ms. Doe will relate positively about the nursing home environment on Monday, Wednesday, and Friday of each week when physically prompted to do so by the Trainer.

Objective 3.2 By 1 July 2004 Ms. Doe will relate positively about the nursing home environment on Monday, Wednesday and Friday of each week when gesturally prompted to do so by the Trainer.

Objective 3.3 By 1 October 2004 Ms. Doe will relate positively about the nursing home environment on Monday, Wednesday and Friday of each week when verbally prompted to do so by the Trainer.

Objective 3.4 By 1 January 2005 Ms. Doe will relate positively about the nursing home environment on Monday, Wednesday and Friday of each week independently.

Goal 4. Reduce Separation Anxieties:

Objective 4.1 Ms. Doe will reduce her incidents of persistent verbalization and somatic complaints about separation from family or attachment figures to five (5) episodes per day per week when physically prompted to do so by the Trainer by 1 April 2004.

Objective 4.2 Ms. Doe will reduce her incidents of persistent verbalization and somatic complaints about separation from her family or attachment figures to three (3) episodes per day per week when gesturally prompted to do so by the Trainer by 1 July 2004.

Objective 4.3 Ms. Doe will reduce her incidents of persistent verbalization and somatic complaints about separation from her family or attachment figures to two (2) episodes per day per week when verbally prompted to do so by the Trainer by 1 October 2004.

Objective 4.4 Ms. Doe will reduce her incidents of persistent verbalization and somatic complaints about separation from her family or attachment figures to zero (0) episodes per day per week independently by 1 January 2005.

Goal 5. Become More Independent.

Objective 5.1 Within three (3) months (1 March 2004) Ms. Doe will board bus to participate in program of community awareness activities each day and on time for the event when physically prompted to do so by the Trainer.

Objective 5.2 Within six (6) months (1 July 2004) Ms. Doe will board bus to participate in program of community awareness activities each day and on time for the event when gesturally prompted to do so by the Trainer.

Objective 5.3 Within nine (9) months (1 October 2004) Ms. Doe will board bus to participate in program of community awareness activities each day and on time for the event when verbally prompted to do so by the Trainer.

Objective 5.4 Within twelve (12) months (1 January 2005) Ms. Doe will board bus to participate in program of community awareness activities each day and on time independently on eight (8) of ten (10) trials.

IV. A Review of Writing Objectives.

Definition:

*Objectives tell in behavioral terms exactly what you want your resident to DO when he or she completes a particular segment of training;

*Objectives are SPECIFIC and GOAL DIRECTED;

*They are OUTCOME – ORIENTED:

*They are TIME – LINKED;

*They have a BEGINNING and COMPLETION DATE;

*They mandate that behavior can and must be OBSERVED, MEASURED, RECORDED and TRACKED;

*They tell HOW LONG;

*They tell HOW MUCH;

*They tell HOW OFTEN;

Example:

Goal: Ms. Doe will adhere to a schedule.

Objective: Within six (6) months (HOW LONG) (1 September 2004) Ms. Doe WILL state the time of day correctly (HOW MUCH) to the minute on eight (8) of ten (10) trials (HOW OFTEN) when verbally instructed to do so by trainer.

V. A Review: Some Examples of Goals and Objectives.

1) Goal: Improve/Maintain Social Skills:

Objective: Ms. Doe will relate positively to others during daily social events on Monday, Wednesday and Friday of each week when verbally prompted to do so by trainer By 1 October 2004.

2) Goal: Improve/Maintain Participation in Activities:

Objective: Ms. Doe will improve her "physical stamina" by walking for fifteen (15) minutes without stopping for rest on every day of week when verbally prompted to do so by trainer by 1 October 2004.

3) Goal: Improve/Maintain Adjustment Skills:

Objective: By 1 October 2004 Ms. Doe will relate positively to others and to nursing home environment on Monday, Wednesday and Friday of each week when verbally prompted to do so by Trainer.

4) Goal: Reduce Separation Anxieties:

Objective: Ms. Doe will reduce her incidents of persistent verbalization and Sematic complaints about separation from family or attachment figures to Five (5) episodes per day per week when physically prompted to do so by the Trainer by 1 April 2004.

5) Goal: Become More Independent:

Objective: Within six (6) months (1 August 2004) Ms. Doe will board bus to participate in community awareness program by herself each day on time for the event when verbally prompted to do so by trainer.

VI. A Review: How Goals and Objectives are Similar.

1) Both emphasize competency and not deviancy;

2) Both are written in positive language;

3) Both reflect sequential and progressive behavior;

4) Both are realistic;

5) Both are understandable to the staff and resident alike.

Goals and Objectives are Different in Three (3) Ways:

1) Objectives describe observable and measurable behavior – goals do not.

2) Objectives are time-linked – goals are not.

3) Objectives are outcome-orientated – goals are not.

CHAPTER SIX

DEVELOPING STRATEGIES

In the preceding chapters emphasis was placed on developing and writing goals and objectives. In review, goals were defined as a road map giving general directions in which the individual activity plan would go while objectives were described as being more detailed and precise statements of what the residents behavior would be like when training was completed. Another important part of the individual therapeutic activity plan is to develop strategies which are even more specific and detailed than objectives. Strategies are the action part of the activity plan. Strategies define for the staff and resident alike what must be done to complete an objective. Strategies state: 1) who will do the training, 2) when the training will be done, and 3) how it will be done. Below are examples of goals, objectives and strategies.

Goal: A goal will always show the general direction of training.

Example: John will develop a friendship with another person.

Objective: An objective will always specify exactly what the residents behavior will be at the end of the training.

Example: John will look at another person during small group sessions with verbal prompts 3 of 5 times on 10 consecutive trials.

Strategy: A strategy will always state who, when, and how resident will meet objective.

Example: The trainer, or his or her designee, will implement task during small group session. If John looks at another person following a verbal prompt on 3 to 5 times on 10 consecutive trials he will be rewarded immediately by the trainer by a pat on the back and a comment of "good job, John - - you looked at another person." Also, he will be rewarded by allowing him to watch television in the evening. However, if he does not respond in a positive manner to the task he will not be rewarded.

Goal: A goal will always show the general direction of training.

Example: John will drink from a glass.

Objective: An objective will always specify exactly what the residents behavior will be at the end of the training.

Example: John will pick up his glass raising it to his mouth with verbal prompts on 3 of 5 times during each meal for 8 consecutive meals.

Strategy: A strategy will always state who, when and how resident will meet objective.

Example: Ms. Hill, LPN will train John during dressing in the morning prior to the breakfast meal. She will give John the verbal command of "John, put on your shirt." If John responds by putting on his shirt, he will be rewarded by Ms. Hill who will say.—"good boy, John—you put on your shirt", giving him an affectionate pat on his back. She will also give him a drink or food of his choice. If he fails to respond to task, he will not be rewarded.

Who is necessary to make a strategy work?

It takes people, a team effort and continuiety to make a strategy work. This is one situation where the interdisciplinary team functions at its best. The team selects an appropriate individual or individuals to assume the responsibility for planning, developing and implementing a strategy or strategies. Then too, the team supervises strategy development and the training of staff members who will be working with the resident or residents. The individual implementing the strategy will almost always be someone who is a staff member already familiar and working with the resident and who has the ability and/or the capacity to be trained in administering behavioral strategies. Trainers will be selected primarily from the direct care staff who knows the resident and who are already working with the resident in the specific areas which need improvement. The strengths and needs list can be extremely important in selecting a trainer by indicating which individual on the staff to whom the resident is most responsive. The supervisors and members of the professional staff who have expertise and experience will generally provide advice, assistance as well as teaching behavioral techniques to the caretakers who have limited knowledge in behavior therapies. This should be an ongoing and never ending process of inservice training. In conclusion the team provides enough support to permit the trainer to carry out the training of the resident without unduly restricting his or her right to formulate a strategy, and to change or modify it. The team should monitor, encourage their training effort, check its progress and reward the trainer with verbal reinforcement.

When developing strategies such as the preceding examples, they can be written in a simple manner or they may be more detailed and complex depending on the nature of the program and task. However, they must address WHO, WHEN, AND HOW training will be done to include the following:

1) The name of the program being taught.

2) The name of the task.

3) The number of steps in the task.

4) The techniques of teaching the tasks.

5) The nature of the assistance provided by the trainer.

Such detailed planning assists the trainer in knowing exactly what to do when working with the resident. It forces the trainer to consider possible barriers which might interfere with the resident being able to pass his or her objective. It helps the trainer to find possible solutions to these barriers. It helps the trainer to become part of the solution and not part of the problem in such areas as transportation, scheduling, space, location, personnel and cooperation of individuals who will be involved in or supporting the training of the residents. The following are examples:

EXAMPLE:

NAME: John Doe

PROGRAM: Dressing

TASK: Put on Shoe

OBJECTIVE: To teach resident to put on his shoe upon request, without discriminating right shoe from left shoe and without lacing.

MATERIALS: A moccasin-type right shoe or right loafer two sizes too large for resident; a tie-type right shoe resident's normal size. Both have laces removed or loosened. A shoehorn (optional).

SETTING: Resident and trainer sitting on floor, resident with socks on and shoes off.

BASELINE: Use normal sized shoe. Place right shoe beside resident's right foot. Trainer touches shoe and says,

"John, put on your shoe."

Do not reinforce a correct response and do not correct an incorrect response. Give no assistance.

TRAINING PROCEDURE

STEP 1:   Use oversized loafer-type shoe. Begin with resident's right heel half-way inside oversized shoe. Trainer assists resident to hold shoe tongue (or top of shoe) up with one hand and to place shoe horn (or index finger of the other hand) down inside the back of the shoe. Trainer says,

"John, put on your shoe,"
and immediately assist resident to push his heel into the shoe.

STEP 2:   Use oversized shoe. Begin with resident's right heel outside oversized shoe, toes inside. Trainer assists resident to hold shoe tongue (or top of shoe) and to use shoehorn or index finger. Trainer says,

"John, put on your shoe,"
and immediately assists resident to push heel into shoe.

STEP 3:   Use oversized shoe. Place oversized right shoe beside resident's right foot. Trainer assists resident to align shoe with front of foot, hold shoe tongue (or top of shoe) and use shoehorn (or index finger). Trainer says,

"John, put on your shoe,"
and immediately assists resident to put toes into shoe and push heel into shoe.

STEP 4:   Terminal Behavior. Use normal-sized loafer or tie-
                          type shoe. Place fitted right shoe beside resident's
                          right foot. Trainer touches shoe and says,

                          "John, put on your shoe." (See Note 1).
                          Give minimal reinforcement and assistance as re-
                          quired.

                          If resident has difficulty with the normal-sized
                          shoe, try putting talcum powder or corn starch
                          on the bottom of sock and inside resident's shoe
                          to help alleviate the difficulty of the sock resisting
                          as it is pushed into the shoe.
                          Once resident has mastered tying and right-left
                          shoe discrimination, these task may also be re-
                          quired as part of resident's putting on his shoes.

HOW to make a strategy work.

This part of developing and implementing a strategy is always the
most challenging aspect of the entire process of writing the residents individual therapeutic activity plan for the activity specialist and his or her staff.
Although there are numerous ways and means of training the Alzheimer
resident, the same approach does not always work for all residents or for
all objectives. Here again reliance upon the team approach to assist with
problem solving will give the trainer several different prospectives and approaches to developing a variety of different teaching strategies which will
increase his or her changes of being successful. Then, too, there are several
general principles to keep in mind when developing any strategy. They
are: 1) all strategies should compliment the task selected to be learned, 2)
compliment the trainers own skills and 3) recognize the strengths of the

resident. However, regardless of the strategy selected, the training should always be selected on the basis that it will assist the resident to become more independent and or to help him or her maintain their skills at its present level of functioning.

When planning how to achieve an objective the following basic principles should be considered. They are:

1) The method of performing the task.

As previously stated there is always a number of ways and means of designing a program and performing a task. Regardless of a program or task chosen, it must be designed in accordance with the residents capabilities. For example:

The nursing home facility in which you were employed as an activity director admitted Mr. John Doe to the Alzheimer's Unit on which you were assigned with a diagnosis of Dementia of the Alzheimer's Type. He also had a history of hypertension, high blood pressure and had recently experienced a mild stroke. During his assessment it was established that he lost many of his self-help and practical living skills. Therefore, the team decided upon a program for Mr. Doe in dressing with a task of putting on his pants.

In developing a dressing strategy of Mr. Doe the team had to determine the best method for him to perform the task. In making their choice they had to consider Mr. Doe's lost skills, his physical limitations caused by his stroke, his current needs and the routines that he would be expected to follow after his training was completed.

Steps in the Task.

Once the method of doing a task was decided upon by the team, the next step was to break the task down into as many small steps as possible. For example, the task of putting on a pair of pants, using the method illustrated earlier, was broken down into the following steps. The team had to keep in mind that if the steps were too large then they might discourage the resident while if they were too small they might tend to bore him. They then numbered the steps and described them in as few words as possible.

EXAMPLE:

PROGRAM: Dressing.

TASK: Putting on pants.

OBJECTIVE: To teach resident, Mr. John Doe to put on his pants upon request, without zipping, snapping, or discriminating front from back. (Use prompts if needed.)

MATERIALS: A pair of pants two sizes too large for him; a pair of pants of normal size for him. Both pair of pants will have elastic waistbands as indicated in each step.

BASELINE: Use normal-sized pants. Mr. Doe sits on edge of bed or chair. Give Mr. Doe his pants. Trainer touches pants and says "Mr. Doe, put on your pants." Do not reinforce any response at this point and time and do not correct in incorrect response.

STEPS:

Step 1. Use oversized pants. Mr. Doe is standing. Begin with oversized pants at Mr. Doe's mid-hip level. Trainer says: "Mr. Doe..put on your pants" and immediately assist Mr. Doe to grasp the waistband (his thumbs hooked over the waistband and his fingers outside, pulling upward) and pull his pants up to his waistline level.

Step 2. Use oversized pants. Mr. Doe is standing. Begin with oversized pants at his knee level. Trainer says: "Mr. Doe, put on your pants." and immediately assist Mr. Doe to grasp waistband (thumb hooked over waistband, fingers outside) and pull pants up from knees to waistline level.

Step 3. Use oversized pants. Mr. Doe is standing. Begin with oversized pants pushed down to his feet, with feet still showing. Trainer says: "Mr. Doe, put on your pants." and immediately assist Mr. Doe to grasp waistband and pull his pants up from feet to waistline level.

Step 4. Use oversized pants. Mr. Doe is sitting on the edge of a chair. Put his feet into leg holes so that the waistband is at residents ankles and pants legs are stretched out. Trainer says, "Mr. Doe, put on your pants," and immediately assist Mr. Doe to lift his right foot and pull up the sides of the right pants leg until his foot is visible. Trainer then assists him to place his foot on the floor. Repeat similar action with the left foot. Mr. Doe should then stand up and pull pants up from feet to waistline level.

Step 5. Use oversized pants. Mr. Doe is sitting on the edge of chair. Give resident his pants. Trainer says, "Mr. Doe, put on your pants," and immediately assist Mr. Doe to grasp waistband (so that leg holes are visible and positioned across from appropriate legs) and then put each leg in the appropriate leg hole. He should then complete action until pants are pulled up to the waistline level.

Step 6. Terminal behavior. Use normal-sized pants. Mr. Doe sits on edge of chair. Give him his pants. Trainer touches pants and says, "Mr. Doe, put on your pants. Trainer will give minimal assistance with reinforcement by patting Mr. Doe on his back and saying, "Good job, Mr. Doe, you did a good job by putting on your pants."

Step 7. Once Mr. Doe has met criteria with oversized pants, repeat the procedure with a pair of pants that fit.

Step 8. Terminal behavior: Use normal-sized pants (pants that fits). Mr. Doe sits on edge of chair. Give him his pants. Trainer touches pants and says, "Mr. Doe, put on your pants." Trainer will give Mr. Doe minimum assistance and reinforcement. If Mr. Doe completes task by pulling his pants up to his waistline level the trainer wills ay, "Good job, Mr. Doe, -- you put on your pants."

The following are some examples of how task(s) are broken down into steps. One of the best ways to break down a task into a number of small steps is to perform the task on oneself and write down all the steps that one can pick out. When tasks are broken down into a number of small steps it benefits both the resident and staff alike. It makes training easier for the staff member doing the training and helps the elderly resident suffering from dementia to be more responsive to the training process.

ACTIVITY TASK

EXAMPLE

Task: Walk Independently.

Steps:

1) Resident able to coordinate erect postural movement of head, trunk and arms with movement of each leg as they move ALTERNATELY through a stance phase and a swing phase to propel the body forward. The trainer will assist using physical, gestural and verbal prompts.

2) Resident ABLE to perform above movements with physical prompting by trainer.

3) Resident ABLE to perform above movements with gestural prompting by trainer.

4) Resident ABLE to perform above movements with verbal prompting by trainer.

5) Resident ABLE to perform above movements independently without assistance from trainer, a stationary object or assistive device.

6) Resident ABLE to walk around assigned walking area with physical prompts from trainer.

7) Resident ABLE to walk around assigned walking area with gestural prompts from trainer.

8) Resident ABLE to walk around assigned walking area with verbal prompting from trainer.

9) Resident ABLE to walk around assigned walking area independently.

10) Program completed when resident is ABLE to walk around assigned walking area independently on three consecutive times during five trials when requested to do so by trainer.

ACTIVITY TASK
EXAMPLE

TASK: DEODORANT USE

Steps:

1) Pick up container.

2) Take cover off.

3) Raise left arm.

4) Spray (or rub) deodorant under arm.

5) Lower arm.

6) Raise right arm.

7) Spray (or rub) under arm.

8) Lower right arm.

9) Replace cover.

10) Return to shelf.

ACTIVITY TASK

EXAMPLE

TASK: PULLOVER SHIRT OR DRESS

STEPS:

1) Picks up the shirt or dress by the hem so that the front of the garment is to the front of the body.

2) Pulls the neck of the shirt or dress over the head.

3) Puts the left arm into the left sleeve of the garment.

4) Puts the right arm into the right sleeve of the garment.

5) Pulls the hem of the shirt or dress down to the normal waist position or below.

ACTIVITY TASK

EXAMPLE

TASK: TABLE MANNERS.

STEPS:

1) Pick up Appropriate Utensil(s) – Resident should be taught to pick up appropriate utensils provided. These utensils could vary depending on the type of food being served. The primary utensils will be a fork and knife.

2) Eats Without Playing in Food – Resident should not manipulate the food in any way other than is necessary for consumption. This includes squeezing food, throwing food, patting food with spoon, mixing up food, putting bread in milk, etc.

3) Eat Correct Size Bites – Control size of bites, model for the resident the right size bite to eat. If the resident eats with a larger bite than you recommended, point out to him/her the appropriate size and use whatever prompts are needed to have him/her eat appropriate sizes. Use prompts as needed.

4) Eat at Normal Rate – The resident is taught to eat at the correct rate. Make a determination of what a normal rate of eating is by u

sing a stop watch if necessary. Then, if the resident dips his/her fork into his food at a rate faster than is appropriate, tell him/her not to dip until you say it is O.K. to, and if he/she needs, you can hold his/her arm at the biceps to control the rate of eating. Use prompts as needed.

5) Eat Neatly – In order to get the resident toe at neatly, he/she should eat slowly and be sure that he/she doesn't dip his/her fork in and get so much food on it that it will fall off. Use prompts as needed.

6) Does Not Eat from Table or Floor – Resident should not eat food from any other surface than the tray/plate, including the table, floor, lap, etc. This also includes food that has been accidentally pushed off the tray/plate or dropped from the spoon.

7) Use Napkin – Whenever the resident gets food on his/her mouth, he/she should use a napkin to wipe it off. Use prompts as needed.

ACTIVITY TASK

EXAMPLE

TASK: USING COMMODE.

STEPS:

1) Goes into bathroom.

2) Pulls clothing up/pants down to knees.

3) Sits on commode.

4) Eliminates successfully.

5) Wipes and cleans self.

6) Stands and pulls clothing down/pants up, adjusting appropriately.

7) Flush commode.

8) Soaps, washes and dry hands.

9) Leaves bathroom appropriately.

I.   A Review of Writing Strategies.

Definition:

Strategies State:

*WHO will do the training;

*WHEN it will be done;

*HOW it will be done.

Strategies is the THIRD PART of the individual program plan. When writing strategies you become even more SPECIFIC than when writing objectives. Example:

Goal: Show more consideration:

Objective: Ms. Doe will let her roommate choose program of her choice on television on Monday, Wednesday and Friday, independently, by 1 June 2004.

Strategy: Always state WHO, WHEN and HOW to meet the criteria of objective. The Charge LPN or Evening Monitor will check room of resident at 7:00 P.M. with Ms. Doe and her roommate. If on Monday, Wednesday, and Friday Ms. Doe has allowed her room-mate to select television program of her choice the Charge Nurse and/or Monitor will grant one (1) extra hour of viewing time to Ms. Doe. However, if she has not, Ms. Doe will not be rewarded by not allowing her to view any program on any television set that evening.

CHAPTER SEVEN

THE INDIVIDUAL THERAPEUTIC ACTIVITY PLAN

The individual program plan is now an established and accepted format for providing services for the resident(s) who live in long term care facilities. The individual program is required by law, and when written and implemented becomes a living breathing legal document. And even more important, it is extremely beneficial and helpful to the resident, their facilities, and to team members alike. It helps, and in reality, forces all members of the team to focus on the residents treatment, promotes continuity of care and accents accountability. It forces team members to define specific need(s) of the individual and presents the resident with tasks that he or she needs to learn, unlearn, relearn, or wants to learn.

The individual program plan is a new concept for the recreational community which up until recent years focused primarily on providing general, leisure – time, and nonspecific activity programming. Developing an individual therapeutic activity plan takes some getting accustomed to and there is usually a lot of anxiety, resistance, and procrastination on the part of the staff citing personnel shortage, a lack of time and scheduling as reasons against it.

However, they are written to take the place of, and not duplicate, much of the paperwork that the staff is required to do and in the long run will save both time and level of work. Like anything new or different, the individual program plan concept takes time to get used to and accept. However, each time a plan is written, the easier the task becomes. In the end, the plan will be done faster and improve in quality than the one done previously. And as a result, the resistance on the part of staff will decrease. After all the purpose of the plan is to teach the resident(s) skills needed to accomplish tasks without assistance. And as they become more independent this will free the trainer and staff up to devote more time to writing and implementing individual program plans with improved goals, objectives, strategies, and methods of evaluation.

The following are examples of formats of an activity assessment, individual therapeutic activity plans and methods for recording data. There are others. In fact, you may want to develop your own. However, regardless of the format used, the plan must contain four basic parts: 1) goals, 2) objectives, 3) strategies and 4) evaluation. And, remember they are required, t hey are helpful to the resident and their families, and they are useful to the staff. They should be developed and written with team participation and input accenting a unique service, a unique body of knowledge, and a unique philosophy on the part of activity personnel.

James W. Ramage Ph.D.

INDIVIDUAL THERAPEUTIC ACTIVITY PLAN
EXAMPLE Page 1

Resident _John Doe_ Age _74_ Record No. _20 01 02_
Date of ITAP _1-1-05_ Date Completed _1-7-05_ Date Implemented _1-10-05_

The persons listed below attended team meeting held on _1-1-05_ for _Mr. John Doe_ for the purpose of developing an individual therapeutic activity plan and doing so with maximum involvement of attending team members, the resident and family members alike. This activity plan was developed individualized, tailored to and written to define, target and address a specific need or needs of _Mr. Doe_ following comprehensive assessments to include behavioral, medical, recreational, social and functional analysis.

The method of implementing plan will consist of resident(s) being rewarded by trainer when exhibiting desired and or appropriate behavior by using verbal, gestural, and physical prompts. Activities will also serve as reinforcers such as sitting in a special chair, going for a ride or walk, watching a movie, etc. In addition, liquids and edibles are also used as reinforcers when approved by medical and dietary staff. The resident(s) will always be given an explanation of why a reward is being given. All progress or lack of it will be documented and reflected in progress notes.

The plan will be implemented by trained and supervised staff in a technically sound, humane and non-intrusive manner as possible in accordance with all legal and ethical standards of society.

Signature	Title
Beatrice Styles, L.P.N.	Nursing Services.
Sue Able, S.S.D.	Social Services.
Kinny Worker, L.C.S.W.	Clinical Social Worker.
Jimmy Shots, R.N.	Nursing Supervisor.
Auto Specialist, M.A.	Communication Specialist.
Lewis South, C.N.A.	Nursing Services.
Psyche Bender, M.A.	Psychological Associate.
Susan Dogood, M.S., A.C.C.	Consultant Activities.
David Action, A.A., ADC.	Activity Director.

100

INDIVIDUAL THERAPEUTIC ACTIVITY PLAN (ITAP)

Name *John Doe*   Date *1-1-05*   Room No. *15*

Resident Participated in Developing Activity Plan: Yes _✓_ No ___ Comments *Able to discuss with team his likes and dislikes*

Family Participated in Developing Plan: Yes _✓_ No __ Comments *His daughter (legal guardian) was able to give good family history.*

Strengths	Needs
Responds to simple questions	*Improve strength in lower extremities*
Follows simple directions	*Improve strength in upper extremities*
Identifies environmental objects	*Improve social skills*
Able to attend to a task	*Reduce aggressive behavior*
Ambulatory	*Reduce inappropriate verbalizations*

Prioritized I Goals	Prioritized II Goals
Reduce aggressive behavior	*Improve social skills*
Reduce inappropriate verbalizations	
Strengthen lower extremities	
Strengthen upper extremities	

Schedule: Days *Monday - Friday* Times *5-7 days @ meals* Trainer(s) *David Action, ADC*

(Circle Assigned Group)

Group A	Group B	Group C
(a) Mild Skill Loss	(a) Moderate Skill Loss	(a) Severe Skill Loss
(b) In Room Activity	(b) In Room Activity	(b) In Room Activity
(c) In Assigned Area	(c) In Assigned Area	(c) In Assigned Area
(d) In Large Group	(d) In Large/Small Group	(d) In Small Group
(e) Other ____	(e) Other *hallway/dining room*	(e) Other ____

Interest, Requirement or Need: (Check Appropriately): Social _✓_ Religious _✓_ Indoor _✓_ Outdoor _✓_ Creative ___ Music ___ Educational ___ Relaxation _✓_ Cognitive _✓_ Esteem Building ___ Exercise _✓_ Outings ___ Self Help Skills _✓_ ADL's _✓_ Psychological _✓_ Other (Explain) *Needs Behavior Reduction plan.*

Special Directions: *Relate to him in a kind but firm manner using physical, gestural and verbal prompting to perform task independently. Reward all desired and positive responses immediately.*

Strategy: (who, when, how) *Trainer will lead training activity by developing, implementing and collecting data on the performance of the above in a safe place in accordance with program. All staff will support and augment training.*

Therapeutic Purpose of Activity: *Reduce inappropriate behavior and strengthen extremities.*

Barrier *Lack of energy*   Solution *Refer to Medical Staff for assessment.*
Barrier *Lack of motivation*   Solution *Refer to Behavioral Health for evaluation.*

Process Evaluation Done: *Strategies examined following each training session.*
Post Evaluation Done: Date ____ Results *will be done when completing each step.*

Approved By: *Susan Bogard, MA, Acc* Completed By: *David Action, ADC*
      Consultant   Title

COMPREHENSIVE ACTIVITY ASSESSMENT
EXAMPLE

NAME: _John Doe_   RECORD NO:_200102_
ROOM NO.:__15__   DATE OF ASSESSMENT _12-10-04_
DATE OF BIRTH:_12-19-30_

I. SENSORY/MOTOR CHARACTERISTICS: CHECK THOSE THAT APPLY:

A. Hearing
    1. Normal
    2. Mild Loss
    3. Moderate Loss ✓
    4. Severe/Profound
B. Speech
    1. Intelligible ✓
    2. Partially Intelligible
    3. Unintelligible
    4. Non-Verbal
    A. Gestures
        1. Points
        2. Nods Head
        3. Uses Facial Expressions
        4. Body Movements
C. Vision
    1. Normal
    2. Limited, Wears Glasses ✓
    3. Limited, Won't Wear Glasses
    4. Blind

II. CHARACTER/PERSONALITY TRAITS:
    A. Shows Perseverance Despite Failure
    B. Shows Self-Confidence
    C. Shows Self-Motivation
    D. Shows Appropriate Emotional Response
    E. Hyperactive
    F. Cheerful
    G. Considerate
    H. Argumentative ✓
    I. Unresponsive
    J. Withdrawn
    K. Disruptive ✓

III. ENVIRONMENTAL AWARENESS:
    A. Self Awareness:
        1. Will Allow Passive Exercise ✓
        2. Can Move Upper Extremities ✓
        3. Can Move Lower Extremities ✓
        4. Will Touch Own Upper Extremities ✓
        5. Will Touch Own Lower Extremities ✓
        6. Can Identify Body Parts Verbally ✓

B. SENSORY STIMULATION/ATTENDING:
   1. Will Touch Different Textures With Hands or Feet   ✓
   2. Will Touch Hot And Cold Objects   ——
   3. Will Rub Own Body Surfaces   ——
   4. Will Allow Someone To Rub Body Parts With Lotion   ✓
   5. Will Rub Own Body Parts With Lotion   ——
   6. Blinks Eye When Confronted By An Object   ✓
   7. Looks At An Object Or Person   ✓
   8. Attends To An Object Or Person   ✓
   9. Tracks Object With Eyes   ✓
   10. Gives Eye Contact On Command   ✓
   11. Follows Simple Commands   ✓
   12. Turns Head To Locate Sound   ✓
   13. Reaches For Source Of Stimulus   ✓
   14. Grasps And Manipulates Objects   ✓
   15. Releases Object To Obtain Another   ✓

C. BODY POSITIONS/PLANES
   1. Suspended Prone - Head, Hands, and Legs
      Are Completely Down   ——
   2. Prone - Lifts And Holds Head Up For 5 Seconds   ——
   3. Prone - Lifts Arms For 5 Seconds   ✓
   4. Prone - Lifts Legs For 5 Seconds   ✓
   5. Turns Head Side To Side   ✓
   6. Prone - Rests On Forearms Raising Head and Chest   ——
   7. Prone - Pushes Up On Hands   ——
   8. Prone - Bears Weight On One Hand   ——
   9. Changes From Prone To Sitting Position   ✓
   10. Rolls Over - Prone To Supine and Back Again   ✓
   11. Sits With Support   ——
   12. Sits Without Support   ✓
   13. Sits And Turns From Side To Side   ✓
   14. Can Stand From A Sitting Position Without Help   ✓
   15. Stands With Assistance   ——
   16. Alternates Feet In Stepping Movement   ✓
   17. Lowers Self From Standing To Sitting Position   ✓
   18. Stands Alone For 1 Minute   ✓
   19. Avoids Objects While Walking   ✓
   20. Walks On Tiptoes   ——
   21. Propells Wheelchair   ——

D. IMMEDIATE SURROUNDINGS:
   1. Knows Location Of Bed And Personal Belongings   ——
   2. Knows How To Go To The Restroom Alone   ✓
   3. Knows Location Of Dining Room   ✓
   4. Learning Staff Members   ——
   5. Knows What Room He/She Resides In   ——
   6. Knows Whereabouts At All Times   ——

VI. RECREATIONAL SKILLS AND INTERESTS:
A. PASSIVE ACTIVITY:
    1. Puts Puzzle Together
    2. Rocks In Rocking Chair
    3. Looks At Magazines And Books
    4. Watches TV and Movies
    5. Enjoys Listening To Music
    6. Can Play Various Card Games
    7. Can Play Checkers and/or Dominoes
    8. Can Play Other Simple Table Games Specify
    9. Enjoys Walks Or Wheelchair Strolls
    10. Enjoys Sitting Outside
    11. Enjoys Cook-Outs/Picnics

B. ARTS AND CRAFTS:
    1. Pastes
    2. Tears Paper
    3. Cuts With Scissors
    4. Paints With Brush
    5. Colors
    6. Scribbles
    7. Draws
    8. Manipulates Clay
    9. Models Recognizable Forms In Clay

C. SPORTS/GAMES ACTIVITIES
    1. Strikes Suspended Object With Items Such
        As A Bat Or Paddle
    2. Catches Ball
    3. Throws Ball
    4. Kicks Ball
    5. Stops Rolling Ball With Feet Or Hands
    6. Hits Ball When Thrown
    7. Can Actively Participate In Individual
    8. Can Actively Participate In Team Or Group Activities,
        Ring Toss, Basketball

D. PHYSICAL FITNESS ACTIVITIES
    1. Can Walk Horizontal Bar
    2. Can Lift Weighed Objects
    3. Can Walk Paralled Bars

E. COMMUNITY OUTINGS
    1. Behavior Is Generally Acceptable
    2. Responds To And Enjoys Events That
        Occur During Outing
    3. Can Talk About And/Or Describe Outing Afterwards
    4. Enjoys Sporting Event
    5. Enjoys Musical Programs Or Concerts
    6. Enjoys Window Shopping
    7. Enjoys Dining Out

IV. SOCIAL RECREATIONAL ACTIVITIES AND SKILLS:
1. Smiles At Social Occasions
2. Greets Others In Social Activity
3. Is Aware Of Activity During Social Recreation Sessional Of Parties
4. Expresses Happiness During Social Activity
5. Will Give Object To Other Who Requests It
6. Will Take Object When Offered To Him/Her
7. Initiates Conversation
8. Responds To Conversation
9. Initiates Personal Contact
10. Stops Activity When Told To Do So
11. Will Show Off In Order To Gain Attention
12. Indicates By Gestures Likes or Dislikes
13. Follows Simple Commands
14. Joins Group Activities
15. Sings
16. Claims and Defends Ownership of Belongings
17. Shares and Takes Turns
18. Resist Interferences In Activities
19. Accepts Termination Of Activity
20. Will Say Please and Thank You
21. Accepts Assistance From Others
22. Seeks Assistance When Needed
23. Offers Assistance
24. Aggressive Against Others
25. Aggressive Against Objects
26. Aggressive To Self
27. Exercises Self - Control
28. Forms Close Personal Relationships
29. Shows Cooperation
30. Onlooker In Activities
31. Friendly Or Affectionate
32. Cries Or Whines
33. Rejects Help, Attention

V. SPIRITUAL HISTORY
1. Is Religious
2. Active Member of Church
3. Member of A Denomination
4. Likes Religious Services
5. Enjoys Religious/Gospel Singing
6. Same Religion As Parents
7. Same Denomination as Parents
8. A Believer In God
9. A Believer In A Higher Power
10. Says Prayer Each Day
11. Prays Before Each Meal
12. Has Had A Spiritual Experience
13. Atheist
14. Agnostic
15. Other (Prefer not to discuss)

F. HOBBIES: List any Hobbies That The Client Is Either
Interested In Or Is Currently Involved In
1. *Sports*
2. *Hunting*
3. *Fishing*
4. *gardening*
5. *Outdoors*

G. MISCELLANEOUS INFORMATION: List Any Pertinent Information
Regarding Recreation Programming That Is Not Covered On This
Assessment - This Could Be Such Information As Allergies, Diet, Etc.
Or Special Talents Or Skills The Client Possesses

1. Diet
2. Allergy
3. Special Talent

VII. DEGREE OF PARTICIPATION:
A. Active
B. Passive   _____
C. Partial   _✓_

VIII. FUNCTIONAL SKILLS:
1. Good Self-Help Skills   _____
2. Good Practical Living Skills   _____
3. Good Grooming Skills   _____
4. Good Dressing Skills   _____
5. Good Basic Readiness Skills   _____
6. Good Dining Skills   _____
7. Good Toileting Skills   _____
8. Good Cognitive Skills   _____
9. Maintains Appropriate Behavior _____
10. Exhibits Appropriate Sexual Behavior _____
11. Makes Appropriate Verbalizations _____

IX. FUNCTIONAL ANALYSIS:
1. Behavior(s) Defined   _✓_
2. Behavior(s) Baselined/Targeted, Tracked and Recorded _✓_
3. Experimental Procedures Done To Change
Targeted Behavior(s)   _✓_
4. Recording Of Behavior Continued And Assessed _✓_
5. Reversal Or Multiple - Baseline Design Implemented
To Measure Behavior To See If Desirable Behavior Is
Being Maintained.   _✓_

X. RECOMMENDATIONS;
1. *Needs To Reduce his Aggression*
2. *Needs to Decrease Inappropriate Verbalizations*
3. *Strengthen Upper and Lower Extremities*

SIGNATURE/JOB TITLE *Joe James, ADC .*
DATE *12-10-04*

BEHAVIOR REDUCTION PLAN

RE: JOHN DOE

I. OBJECTIVE

To reduce the rate of his aggression (striking) and inappropriate verbalizations (sexually related subject matter).

II. METHOD

This program stipulates that Mr. Doe will receive verbal praise every hour for the absence of aggressive episodes in addition to being allowed to listen to music for 15 minutes after the evening meal (supper) if he has been aggressive that day. Aggressive behavior is addressed using verbal or physical redirection and, if necessary, removal to a quiet area for 5 minutes. Observations of Mr. Doe's typical behavior suggests that praise and attention are largely responsible for motivating the improvement he has exhibited over the past month and should continue to constitute the primary reinforcement. In addition, it is expected that attention he receives when disruptive—especially attention from females he is attracted to—appears to be incidentally reinforcing his disruptive episodes. Therefore, alterations to the procedures for maladaptive contingencies will stipulate that minimal attention be used to intervene when necessary.

During Mr. Doe's staffing, it was also recommended that a behavioral strategy to address "Inappropriate Verbalizations" be developed.

III. DEFINITIONS

1. Aggression – striking, spitting, scratching, pinching, biting and grabbing others, or attempting any of these.

2. Inappropriate Verbalizations – saying things comprising situational inappropriate subject matter (usually sexually related).

IV. MALADAPTIVE TARGET BEHAVIORS

A. Aggression: The following contingencies will be implemented with no extra verbalizations and with minimal eye contact. Please ensure that no audiences are allowed to observe lest Mr. Doe be accidentally reinforced for being aggressive.

1. Say, "Stop, John" in a firm, loud voice.

2. If necessary, physically interrupt the behavior and prompt him instead to exhibit an activity appropriate to the current program or activity.

3. If he continues, place him in a chair facing away from the group until he is calm for 2 minutes. If necessary, use the minimal amount of hands-on contact necessary to prevent him from leaving the chair.

4. After he completes 2 minutes of calm, prompt him to resume his normal activity.

5. If Mr. Doe continues to be aggressive, remove him from group to quite area or to his room.

6. After he completes 5 minutes of calm, prompt him to return to group.

7. If Mr. Doe remains aggressive after steps 1 thru 6 have been repeated four times, a professional will be consulted to determine further action.

B. Inappropriate Verbalizations

Whenever Mr. Doe exhibits an example of inappropriate verbalizations:

1. Say, "Stop, John" in a firm, loud voice.

2. If Mr. Doe continues, place him in a chair facing away from the group until he is calm for 2 minutes. If necessary, use the minimal amount of hands-on control necessary to prevent him from leaving the chair.

3. After he is calm for 2 minutes, prompt him to resume his normal activity.

4. If he again exhibits inappropriate verbalizations, repeat steps 1, 2, & 3, as many times as needed with consultation from professional for further instructions.

NOTE: Frequent episodes of inappropriate verbalizations is a good indicator that Mr. Doe needs more attention than he is receiving.

Therefore, make sure that any example of appropriate behavior he exhibits is noticed and appropriately praised.

V. DATA COLLECTION

All incidents of inappropriate behavior of aggression and inappropriate verbalizations will be documented. Use of verbal direction and separation from the group will be documented.

VI. STAFF RESPONSIBILITIES

The group leader or assigned relief, assigned program services staff, and any inserviced staff are responsible for implementing the program as written, recording episodes of adaptive and maladaptive behaviors and the occurrence reinforcement.

The supervisor is responsible for ensuring that the program in the group notebook remains with the group at all times, the required positive reenforcers are available, and monitoring to ensure that the program is implemented as needed and data collected, and forwarding data to be recorded on a daily basis.

The supervisor is also responsible for providing inservice training to all relevant staff, monitoring to ensure the program is implemented, correctly. Formal monitoring will be done on a weekly basis. The supervisor is also responsible for evaluating the effectiveness of the program and initiating revisions/changes as needed.

The supervisor in conjunction with the team is responsible for monitoring to ensure the program is implemented, necessary supplies are available, data collected, and that the program is effective.

VII. MEDICATION:

The team feels that Mr. Doe would benefit from Neuroleptic Medication (Buspar) due to the following behaviors: 1) aggression and 2) inappropriate verbalization of a sexual nature. The team feels that in this case the benefits of the medication far outweigh the risks.

Reduction Criteria: Further reduction will be considered by the team when Mr. Doe's behavior (rate of aggression and inappropriate verbalizations) meets the criteria of the prescribed goals and objectives.

Behavior Plan Prepared By _Susan Osgood, ACC_

Behavior Plan Approved By _David Action, ADC._

INDIVIDUAL THERAPEUTIC ACTIVITY PLAN
GOALS AND OBJECTIVES
EXAMPLE

Resident _John Doe_ Program _Behavior problem_
Goal 1 _Reduce aggression_

Objective 1.1 _Mr. Doe will reduce his incidents of aggression to three (3) or less occurrences per month by 03-31-05._

Date Started _1-10-05 (JJ)_ Date Ended _3-29-05 (JJ)_
Reason Obj. Ended _Completed Objective (JJ)_
Rationale For Change _____
Signature of Trainer _Joe Jones, ADC_

Objective 1.2 _Mr. Doe will reduce his incidents of aggression to two (2) or less occurrences per month by 05-31-05._

Date Started _4-1-05 (JJ)_ Date Ended _5-31-05 (JJ)_
Reason Obj. Ended _Completed Objective (JJ)_
Rationale For Change _____
Signature of Trainer _Joe Jones, ADC._

Objective 1.3 _Mr. Doe will reduce his incidents of aggression to one (1) or less occurrences per month by 08-31-05._

Date Started _6-1-05 (JJ)_ Date Ended _7-31-05 (JJ)_
Reason Obj. Ended _Completed Objective (JJ)_
Rationale For Change _____
Signature of Trainer _Joe Jones, ADC_

Objective 1.4 _____

_____

Date Started _____ Date Ended _____
Reason Obj. Ended _____
Rationale For Change _____
Signature of Trainer _____

Objective: 1.5 _____

_____

Date Started _____ Date Ended _____
Reason Obj. Ended _____
Rationale For Change _____
Signature of Trainer _____

James W. Ramage Ph.D.

INDIVIDUAL THERAPEUTIC ACTIVITY PLAN
GOALS AND OBJECTIVES
EXAMPLE

Resident _John Doe_   Program _Behavior Problem_
Goal 2 _Decrease episodes of inappropriate verbalizations_

Objective 2.1 _Mr. Doe will have no more than 14 episodes of inappropriate verbalizations for five (5) consecutive days by 1-31-05._
Date Started _1-18-05 (JJ)_   Date Ended _1-28-05 (JJ)_
Reason Obj. Ended _Completed Objective (JJ)_
Rationale For Change _____
Signature of Trainer _Joe Jones, ADC._

Objective 2.2 _Mr. Doe will have no more than ten (10) episodes of inappropriate verbalizations for five (5) consecutive days by 3-31-05._
Date Started _3-1-05 (JJ)_   Date Ended _3-31-05 (JJ)_
Reason Obj. Ended _Completed Objective (JJ)_
Rationale For Change _____
Signature of Trainer _Joe Jones, ADC._

Objective 2.3 _Mr. Doe will have no more than five (5) episodes of inappropriate verbalizations for five (5) consecutive days by 5-31-05._
Date Started _4-5-05 (JJ)_   Date Ended _5-28-05 (JJ)_
Reason Obj. Ended _Completed Objective (JJ)_
Rationale For Change _____
Signature of Trainer _Joe Jones, ADC._

Objective 2.4 _Mr. Doe will have no more than five (5) episodes of inappropriate verbalizations for ten (10) consecutive days by 6-31-05._
Date Started _6-1-05 (JJ)_   Date Ended _6-30-05 (JJ)_
Reason Obj. Ended _Completed Objective (JJ)_
Rationale For Change _____
Signature of Trainer _Joe Jones, ADC._

Objective 2.5 _____
_____
Date Started _____ Date Ended _____
Reason Obj. Ended _____
Rationale For Change _____
Signature of Trainer _____

114

INDIVIDUAL THERAPEUTIC ACTIVITY PLAN
GOALS AND OBJECTIVES
EXAMPLE

Resident _John Doe_   Program _Motor Activities_

Goal 3 _Strengthen lower extremities_

Objective 3.1 _Within three (3) months, Mr. Doe will walk to the dining room to dine. One (1) time each day on five (5) of seven (7) days with physical prompts from the trainer._

Date Started _1-18-05 (JJ)_   Date Ended _1-28-05 (JJ)_

Reason Obj. Ended _Objective Completed. (JJ)_

Rationale For Change _____

Signature of Trainer _Joe Jones, ADC_

Objective 3.2 _Within three (3) months, Mr. Doe will walk to the dining room to dine two (2) times each day on five (5) of seven (7) days with gestural prompts from the trainer._

Date Started _2-1-05_   Date Ended _2-28-05 (JJ)_

Reason Obj. Ended _Objective Completed. (JJ)_

Rationale For Change _____

Signature of Trainer _Joe Jones, ADC_

Objective 3.3 _Within three (3) months, Mr. Doe will walk to the dining room to dine three (3) times each day on five (5) of seven (7) days with gestural and verbal prompts from the trainer._

Date Started _3-1-05 (JJ)_   Date Ended _3-31-05 (JJ)_

Reason Obj. Ended _Objective Completed. (JJ)_

Rationale For Change _____

Signature of Trainer _Joe Jones, ADC_

Objective 3.4 _Within three (3) months, Mr. Doe will walk to the dining room to dine three (3) times each day on five (5) of seven (7) days independently when time is announced to eat is announced._

Date Started _4-4-05 (JJ)_   Date Ended _4-29-05 (JJ)_

Reason Obj. Ended _Objective Completed. (JJ)_

Rationale For Change _____

Signature of Trainer _Joe Jones, ADC_

Objective 3.5 _____

_____

Date Started _____ Date Ended _____

Reason Obj. Ended _____

Rationale For Change _____

Signature of Trainer _____

James W. Ramage Ph.D.

INDIVIDUAL THERAPEUTIC ACTIVITY PLAN
GOALS AND OBJECTIVES
EXAMPLE

Resident *John Doe*   Program *Motor Activities*
Goal 4 *Strengthen upper extremities*

Objective 4.1 *Within three (3) months Mr. Doe will lift a 2 lb. bean bag with both hands while standing upright from his thigh to his waistline, one (1) time every 15 seconds for one (1) minute, on 5 of 7 days with physical assistance from trainer.*
Date Started *4-5-05 (JJ)*   Date Ended *4-7-05 (JJ)*
Reason Obj. Ended *Program too difficult (JJ)*
Rationale For Change *Bean bag too heavy.*
Signature of Trainer *Joe Jones, ADC*

Objective 4.2 *Within three (3) months Mr. Doe will lift a # lb. bean bag with both hands while standing upright, from his thigh to his waistline one (1) time every 15 seconds for one (1) minute, on 5 of 7 days with physical assistance from trainer.*
Date Started *4-11-05 (JJ)*   Date Ended *4-29-05 (JJ)*
Reason Obj. Ended *Objective Completed. (JJ)*
Rationale For Change
Signature of Trainer *Joe Jones, ADC*

Objective 4.3 *Within three (3) months Mr. Doe will lift a # lb. bean bag with both hands while standing upright from his thigh to his waistline 2 times every 15 seconds for one (1) minute, on 5 of 7 days with gestural prompts from trainer.*
Date Started *5-2-05 (JJ)*   Date Ended *5-31-05 (JJ)*
Reason Obj. Ended *Completed Objective (JJ)*
Rationale For Change
Signature of Trainer *Joe Jones, ADC*

Objective 4.4 *Within three (3) months Mr. Doe will lift a # lb. bean bag with both hands while standing upright from his thigh to his waistline 3 times every 15 seconds for one (1) minute, on 5 of 7 days with verbal prompts from trainer.*
Date Started *6-1-05 (JJ)*   Date Ended *6-30-05 (JJ)*
Reason Obj. Ended *Objective Completed. (JJ)*
Rationale For Change
Signature of Trainer *Joe Jones, ADC*

Objective 4.5 *Within three (3) months Mr. Doe will lift a 1 lb. bean bag with both hands while standing upright from his thigh to his waistline 5 times every 15 seconds for one (1) minute, on 5 of 7 days independently.*
Date Started *7-1-05 (JJ)*   Date Ended *7-29-05 (JJ)*
Reason Obj. Ended *Objective Completed. (JJ)*
Rationale For Change
Signature of Trainer *Joe Jones, ADC*

116

ASSESSMENT OF PROGRESS
EXAMPLE

Resident: *John Doe*   Date of ITAP *1-1-05*
PROGRESS MADE SINCE LAST INDIVIDUAL THERAPEUTIC ACTIVITY
PLAN (ITAP) MEETING

Date	Goal/Obj.#	Program Name	Begun	Ended	Progress
1-10-05	1 - 1.1	Reduce Aggression	1-10-05	3-29-05	Completed objective
1-10-05	2 - 2.1	Decrease PTA Verbalizations	1-10-05	1-28-05	Completed objective
1-10-05	3 - 3.1	Motor Activities	1-10-05	1-28-05	Completed objective
1-10-05	4 - 4.1	Motor Activities	4-5-05	4-7-05	ENDED - Raised O. to difficult.
1-10-05	4 - 4.2	Motor Activities	4-11-05	4-29-05	Objective Completed

CHAPTER EIGHT

THE TRAINING PROCESS

It is difficult to operate effective therapeutic activity programs with large numbers of elderly residents without using behavior management principles and procedures. There are always some individuals who will not cooperate, or who will become disruptive from time to time. However, it is possible, although difficult, to deal with most of these kinds of behavior problems. In attempting to increase the residents cooperativeness and decrease their destructive behavior the interdisciplinary team should develop therapeutic activity plans which are based on sound behavioral philosophy, techniques and principles.

The purpose of developing activity plans based on behavior principles is to teach the resident new skills or maintain existing ones, to reduce inappropriate behavior, to facilitate the occurrence of behavior under appropriate conditions, and to maintain appropriate behavior. The behavior model strengthens the activity plan by insuring that it is therapeutic in that behavior modification is a systemic application of the principles of operant conditioning. Its approach to therapy focuses on objective, observable and measurable behaviors. It addresses behaviors that usually occur first and are later modified or changed by the presentation of some type of stimulus (a re-enforcer). It promotes accountability.

Individual therapeutic activity plans are concerned with the management of behavior of residents suffering from dementia in long term facilities. Their behavior is generally characterized by aggressive acts towards themselves or others, bizarre forms of stereotyped or sexual behavior, temper tantrums and/or violent outbursts of anger, and negativism or general refusal to cooperate. When confronted with such inappropriate behavior, the team members should concern themselves with how to increase the residents cooperativeness and decrease their inappropriate behavior. At this point it is vital that team members define and decide on accelerator techniques and decelerator procedures. Otherwise, the effectiveness of the activity program being developed and implemented will be compromised.

The team should concern themselves with how to use accelerator techniques and decelerator procedures to make the resident more cooperative and how to begin to control his or her inappropriate behavior. The team members should consider also how to use reinforcement procedures and decelerator techniques to prevent the behavior from occurring. Consideration is given to such things as loss of privileges, time out, redirection, required relaxation, over correction, and positive reinforcement to manage his or her inappropriate behavior. And finally, a program plan should then be developed and implemented which will keep the resident actively involved in training in self-help, practical living skills (ADLs), educational programs and interesting activities throughout his or her waking hours.

The challenges of the activity specialist then, with input from team members, is to develop therapeutic programs which target and eliminate the causes of the residents undesirable behavior. This should be done by introducing activity programs that utilize reinforcement procedures as well as scheduling interesting activities which are designed to eliminate inappropriate behavior. The activity specialist begins, in this manner, for both humanitarian and economic reasons. From a humanitarian point of view, the resident should not be subjected to abnormal conditions that cause his or her to act in bizarre or disruptive ways. From an economic point of view, this is the simplest and least expensive way to manage behavior.

If the activity specialist is going to develop an activity plan which is going to target and eliminate the causes of undesirable behavior, he or she needs to know those things that cause the resident to exhibit undesirable behavior. These causes come from two sources), 1) from external causes outside the resident and 2) from internal causes inside the resident. See Table 1.

TABLE I

CONDITIONS THAT CAUSE UNDESIRABLE
BEHAVIOR TO OCCUR

External Causes Outside the Resident	Internal Causes Inside the Resident
1) Difficult Tasks	1) A Need For Attention
2) Interrupting Activity	2) Curiosity
3) Bullying or Teasing	3) A Need For Physical Activity
4) Excessive Heat or Cold	4) Sex Drive
5) A Lack of Visual, Auditory, or Tactile Stimulation (Boredom)	5) Hunger and Thirst
6) Excessive Visual, Auditory, or Tactile Stimulation (excitement)	6) Fatigue

As Table 1 indicates, there are at least six (6) external outside causes of undesirable behavior –things that make a resident angry and irritable or make him or her feel discouraged and hopeless. These are first, difficult tasks at which the resident cannot succeed. They frustrate the resident and make him or her both angry and discouraged about trying to accomplish things. Second, being interrupted when he or she is attempting to accomplish something. Many residents are extremely compulsive about continuing with an activity until it has been completed. If they are interrupted, they become upset and angry. Third, being bullied and teased by another resident. This makes a resident upset, and he or she, in turn, may attack someone else or become destructive, or they may simply lose interest and withdraw from all activities. Fourth, if the resident is too hot, or too cold they may become irritable, agitated and uncontrollable. Fifth, if the resident is bored, has nothing to do, he or she may become irritable and results in them losing interest in everything around them and can promote self-stimulatory behavior such as rocking or slapping themselves, and sixth, being over-stimulated by too many people, noise, and too much excitement going on around them can be extremely upsetting to residents or make them withdraw or result in them behaving in a number of strange and weird ways such as disrobing, trying to elope, masturbating, yelling, exposing themselves, or making strange noises, verbal, or physical threats.

Also, there are six (6) internal causes that go on inside a person that can result in undesirable behavior. First, there is the need for attention. People need recognition for being worthwhile individuals. When they are unable to get recognition for behaving appropriately, they begin to act inappropriately, which invariable gets them the attention they are seeking. Second, people are by nature curious. When they don't have frequent opportunities to satisfy their curiosity, it increases and they are more likely to "get into mischief". Third, everyone has a need for frequently scheduled vigorous physical activities. When they don't get appropriate exercise, they become restless, fidgety, irritable, and even hyperactive. Fourth, people have an overwhelming need to satisfy their sexual needs and or drive. If it cannot be satisfied in socially appropriate sexual ways, many will engage in socially inappropriate sexual activities. Fifth, when people become too hungry or too thirsty, they become irritable and take their frustrations out by expressing anger toward others.

And Sixth, when residents are too tired or exhausted, they become irritable and often express their anger and frustrations toward others.

The primary way to eliminate these causes of undesirable behaviors is to develop and implement activity programs for residents that will eliminate these conditions. The Activity Specialist should, based on the residents needs, schedule a full day of therapeutic activities for each resident that are interesting and/or stimulating. The team should find worthwhile activities for him or her to do at which he or she can succeed, so his or her craving for attention will be satisfied normally. Then the resident will not be bored which is often a problem in nursing home facilities. The resident will, as a result feel wanted, appreciated and will be more responsive to training. The resident who is warm enough, cool enough, is not too tired, and not too thirsty, and who is not being bullied by his peers will develop a more positive attitude and as a result be more receptive to training.

Once the conditions that cause undesirable behavior has been eliminated the Activity Specialist should develop and implement a plan which will keep the resident actively involved in training throughout his or her waking hours. The plan should involve the resident in self-help, practical living skills, educational programs and in meaningful activities.

An example of how such a schedule should be planned is as follows: The resident gets up in the morning and gets him or herself ready to face the day. Since he or she performs the same sequence each morning, in toileting, bathing, grooming, undressing, dressing, and dining, the

Activity Specialist can and should plug into, develop and implement programs in each of these areas. As the resident participates in specifically designed activities in each one of those areas he or she is rewarded with verbal praise for appropriate responses and performances in targeted tasks. And these programs can be repeated throughout the day during the noon and evening meals and at bedtime seven days a week as these activities are tasks that the resident participates in routinely each day.

When the resident finishes breakfast he or she can be scheduled to participate in such programming as picking up and cleaning his or her room, and bed-making during which time he or she receives reinforcement through verbal praise for appropriate responses for a job well done. And then, the resident can be scheduled to participate in various recreational activities which meet a therapeutic need, is interesting and challenging, and which afford him or her to burn up a considerable amount of excess energy. Such participation gives the resident an opportunity to participate in therapeutic activities throughout his or her waking day and up until he or she goes to bed seven days a week.

The evening meal presents the Activity Specialist with another opportunity to involve the resident in training again teaching appropriate dining skills. And following dinner the activity specialist can schedule the resident in meaningful recreational activities such as television, movies, arts and crafts. And finally, at bedtime, toileting, grooming and dressing skills can be taught again. Such a schedule can be repeated daily seven days a week.

It has been established that everything that a resident does, during the day and up until the time he or she goes to bed, can be made a therapeutic activity program. And now emphasis must be placed on how the Activity Specialist communicates with the resident to get the resident to be an active participant in the activity program which he or she has designed and implemented. The following are examples of communication models which might be considered.

Any new or strange treatment system takes time to implement. Therefore, good communication techniques are vital. And because the aim is to help the resident build and/or maintain his or her skill level it is important to be consistent in what he or she does and what they want the resident to do during the treatment process. Therefore, it is imperative that all staff members and healthcare personnel get on the same page as the treatment plan is implemented. The Activity Specialist providing care on the unit where the resident resides should relate to all staff members how to treat the resident as a whole or total person. In order to accomplish this, one must consider the mental, as well as the physical, social, and spiritual needs of the resident. One method of communication which is useful in accomplishing this is "Attitude Therapy". This method emphasizes that all service providers be inserviced on which attitude will be used when interacting with the resident during each shift. It also includes the family or friends who visit or takes the resident on community outings or for a home visit. The therapeutic attitudes are described as follows:

1. **Kind firmness:** The staff will use "kind firmness" when the resident is depressed or uncooperative.

2. **No Demand:** "No demand" is used with the resident who is out of control.

3. **Active friendliness:** Is used by the staff with the withdrawn, and apathetic resident.

4. **Passive friendliness:** Used with the suspicious resident.

5. **Matter-of-fact:** Used with those residents who are manipulative, seductive, or with these residents in the early (near normal) stages of Dementia.

In addition, the use of prompts when training is extremely important in communicating effectively with the resident to make a point or get a message across. Therefore, when training the activity specialist should use the following prompt sequences and codes during the treatment process.

```
┌─────────────────────────────────────────────────────────┐
│           PROMPT SEQUENCE AND CODES                      │
├─────────────────────────────────────────────────────────┤
│  I.   MEANS DID IT INDEPENDENTLY                          │
│  V.   MEANS DID IT WITH VERBAL PROMPTS                    │
│  G.   MEANS DID IT WITH GESTURAL PROMPTS                  │
│  P.   MEANS DID IT WITH PHYSICAL PROMPTS                  │
│  M.   MEANS DID IT WITH MANIPULATIVE PROMPTS              │
├─────────────────────────────────────────────────────────┤
│  +OR YES MEANS DID IT THE WAY THE PROGRAM SAID            │
│  TO DO IT                                                 │
│  -OR NO MEANS DID NOT DO IT THE WAY THE                   │
│  PROGRAM SAID TO DO IT                                    │
│    ("Y" OR "N" MAY ALSO BE USED TO COUNT                  │
│  RESPONSES)                                               │
└─────────────────────────────────────────────────────────┘
```

The teaching or training of residents with dementia poses many challenges for the Activity Specialist. Unacceptable behaviors and memory problems make it extremely difficult to provide care and behavior management to these residents. These behaviors can cause embarrassment, frustration, and exhaustion in individuals attempting to provide care. The Activity Specialist will probably need to explore what works best for him or her and the impaired resident with whom they are working. Listed below are some known problem areas encountered in residents with dementia and some suggestions, techniques and strategies for communicating with and dealing with them. These strategies will help reduce the stress level and assist the specialist in his or her training with residents who exhibit these behaviors. One of the most important skills that the Activity Specialist must learn in working with these residents is communication which requires patience, understanding, acceptance and respect for their pace of learning.

I.   Communication Problems (Both Verbal and Non-verbal).

    A. Make eye contact; hold and maintain his or her attention.

    B. Speak in a slow, deliberate, distinct and clear manner.

    C. Do not yell. Instead speak in a loud but firm voice. Check to see if resident has a hearing problem.

    D. Use simple words.

    E. Make short sentences.

    F. Rephrase thoughts in different ways if the resident does not seem to understand.

    G. Avoid strange accents. They may increase the resident's difficulty in understanding and participating in a conversation.

    H. Monitor the tone and level of your voice when talking to the resident. Use written messages, gestures, pantomime and pictures to make your point.

    I. Use non-verbal cues like grin, smile, or nod. Can be more important than verbal. Write message if necessary to help resident understand.

    J. Do not talk or act around the resident as if he or she is not present.

    K. Construct your method of conversation to match that of the resident. If the resident can respond only with a yes or no, then ask yes or no questions.

L. Be an active listener. If you don't understand, have resident repeat or guess at what the resident is attempting to say.

M. Use humor or sarcasm carefully. They may be offended.

N. Maintain a reassuring and calm manner.

O. Use eye contact, face resident – touch, feeling, rubbing and stroking can all be important.

P. Avoid discussing topics the resident can no longer remember.

Q. Encourage resident to talk about familiar places, interests, past experiences.

II.   Memory Loss, Orientation.

A. Use clocks, calendars, pictures.

B. Use consistent, predictable routines to reduce confusion.

C. Repeat instructions often.

D. Keep important objects and belongings in same place.

E. Use simple directions.

F. Begin conversation with patient by identifying first the resident by name and then oneself.

G. Reduce competing stimulation such as radio and television.

III.   Behavior Problems.

A. Resident to resident problems.

1. Interrupt quickly.

2. Remove the residents from each others space.

3. After residents have calmed down explain to each why you did this using facts only – not guilt.

B. When resident does something wrong.

1. Remove resident from the situation.

2. Redirect their interest in another direction. Remember distraction and redirection can be valuable tools in behavior management.

C. Avoid using isolation as a means of controlling behavior. Isolation leads to increased confusion.

D. Leave the resident alone if he or she lets you know that they are non-receptive.

Tell them that you understand why they don't want to talk or to participate in an activity and that you will be back later. Try again later.

E. If the resident isn't cooperative – *do not force him or her.*

1. Forcing a resident against his or her will only increases disruptive behavior.

2. Try again later.

3. Have a different staff member try.

4. Remember Dementia residents are changeable – their moods can and often changes quickly.

F. When attempting to modify behaviors, note successes and failures on chart so that all personnel on the staff can share and insure consistency in providing care.

G. Treat the resident with dignity and respect at all times. Remember increased self-esteem reduces behavior problems.

H. If you want the resident to go somewhere:

1. Approach him or her from the front, and slowly reach for their hand.

2. Identify yourself and tell the resident where you are going and the reason.

3. Avoid pushing them from behind or from the side. This will increase disruptive behavior.

I. Night Restlessness.

1. Try to reduce daytime naps.

2. Try to keep resident busy or busier during the daytime.

3. At night, convey feelings of security and comfort.

   a. back rubs

   b. embraces

   c. keep a night light on

J. Be aware of your own responses to a situation.

1. Our responses can make a situation worse.

2. Human responses to frustration is normal.

3. Some common reactions of staff

   a. Inconsistent responses

   b. Hostility

   c. Fear

   d. Avoidance of resident

   e. Cold, frigid interaction and/or courtesies

f. Rejection.

K. Dementia residents are extremely sensitive to our mental and emotional reactions. They are more likely to perceive of emotional behavior and responses to them than to understand our spoken words.

L. Learn to be patient and put yourself in the resident's shoes.

1. Reinforce the resident's feelings of belonging in your facility.

a. Use their name every time you see them.

b. Reassure them that this is their home and that you are their friend.

2. Use gestures and touching them as much as possible.

a. Some residents may not understand your words and may respond to a smile or pat on the back.

3. Assaultive Behavior.

a. Causes for verbal or physical violence

1. Confused and disoriented residents are easily frustrated.

2. Simple stresses may frighten or add to confusion.

3. They cannot comprehend the intentions of others.

b. By removing the cause you will usually remove the behavior.

1. Remember the most confused, demented resident is still a human being and, therefore, all human behavior is meaningful and purposeful.

2. The reason for the behavior may be logical to them even

if it may not make sense to us.

3. Look not only at the behavior, but more importantly look for the cause and, if possible, at what it may mean.

4. Do not rush a violent resident with a group of staff members. This usually adds to his or her unacceptable behavior.

And finally, the utilization of augmentative communications should not be overlooked when exploring a way and means of communicating with the Alzheimer's resident. This method should be included because augmentative communication is a substitute or supplemental means of communicating with the resident when the normal process of communicating verbally (speaking) is damaged or absent. Since a communication system is a means of conveying thoughts, ideas, and feelings (examples: speech, manual sign language, Rebus symbols, and gestures). The following methods of augmentative communication should be considered:

1) Indirect/Direct Stimulation

A. Tell or describe activities or movements person is doing

B. Label and tell about objects or things they are manipulating

C. Label and describe objects or things they see in their environment.

D. If verbal ask questions and have them tell about their activities or tasks; likes; dislikes; foods they eat; toileting, grooming, dressing, dining or bathing activities, etc. The list of things to talk about is endless.

Examples of Indirect and Direct Stimulation: Someone putting on a shoe.

Look, here are *your shoes.*

Your shoes are *black.*

You wear shoes on *your feet.*

These are *your feet.*

Watch me put *your shoes* on *your feet.*

There *your shoes* are on *your feet.*

You are *wearing your shoes* on *your feet.*

Additional:

I am *wearing my shoes* on *my feet.*

My shoes are the color *red.*

I tie my shoes with *shoelaces.*

TEACHING A SPOON

Look, this is a spoon.

You use a spoon to eat.

You use a spoon to eat your food.

You eat soup, ice cream, cereal, etc. with a spoon.

Additional:

You eat your peas with a spoon.

You eat your food with a spoon.

Current emphasis is to continue to enhance existing receptive and expressive language skills, while providing appropriate communications systems designed to meet individuals needs and abilities.

Types of Systems:

Verbal = normal process of speaking

Nonverbal = *Gestural* = use of body movements

Manual Sign Language = use of hands and arms in conjunction to facial expressions

Augmentative – supplemental, assistative or a substitute

A. Pictures

B. Rebus Symbols – pictorial symbols

C. Bliss Symbols l- line drawings

D. Orthographic – Alphabet

E. Traditional Orthography written

F. Manual sign language/gestures

Regardless of type of communication system, take into account:

A. Tone of voice

B. Facial expression

C. Body stance/posture – body language

D. Rate of speech

E. Content and length of speech

F. Prompts – verbal, physical, gestural, modeling, manual, etc.

In conclusion, it is important for the Activity Specialist to have more than a basic understanding of the preceding techniques and strategies. By possessing a good knowledge base of these strategies, interventions, modes of communication, and suggestions, the specialist will generally sharpen his or her focus on understanding dementia and the behavior associated with Alzheimer's disease.

Therefore, working with those strategies on a day to day basis will help the specialist define what the resident can and cannot do, what they like and dislike, what staff members, relatives and significant others are available to help, what the staff would like the resident to accomplish, and what the resident would like to do. Further, applying these suggestions and interventions provides the specialist with an opportunity to begin to think in terms of the residents strengths and needs, and begin to think of additional goals and objectives on which the resident needs to work. It also helps the staff realize the importance of the need to implement a team approach to problem solving to insure continuity of care.

Then, too, a staff which is familiar with these strategies helps the resident to develop a trust with the specialist who is an active participant in his or her habilitation. It will, if his or her environment seems safe and secure and the specialist seems competent and consistent in his or her demands, help the resident develop a sense of belonging, reducing his or her level of anxiety, stress, and inappropriate behavior. It will help everyone involved in the habilitative process deal with the residents behavior in the most humane and consistent manner possible.

CHAPTER NINE

EVALUATION

The evaluation component is a necessary and important element of any treatment plan. It is important for a number of reasons such as accreditation, licensure and funding to name a few. However, perhaps the most important function of the evaluation process is to provide the trainer and team members with information which when analyzed will provide them with a base of knowledge which will let them know whether the strategies for implementing the program are working and whether the goals and objectives are being met or not. Evaluation of a program provides the trainer with proof of whether quality service is being provided for the resident and whether the program justifies the time, energy and effort that went into the planning, developing, and implementing the program.

Also, evaluation provides the trainer with the opportunity to focus on, analyze, and utilize the behavioral data obtained during the evaluation process and to examine the prescribed treatment goals, objectives and strategies to see if they meet the following criteria: 1) is the program simple, specific, and doable, 2) does the program reflect a team approach and continuity of care, 3) does it address the individual and specific needs of the resident, 4) does it reflect team planning and input,

5) has the program been evaluated and reevaluated, and 6) does the plan reflect changes, modification, or adjustments as needed.

Then too, evaluation gives the trainer and team members alike the opportunity to seek and depend on empirical data pertaining to the residents plan of treatment rather than on vague subjective statements by others. It motivates the trainer too, during the evaluation, to reexamine key and important questions about the residents plan such as: 1) is the use of social re-enforcers being utilized since they are the easiest to implement and the most likely to last, 2) has the plan, goals, objectives, strategies, been discussed with the residents family and with significant others, 3) are the re-enforcers being used something highly desirable, 4) is the resident being reinforced immediately following an appropriate response, and 5) when reinforcement is given has something tangible been paired with social praise? For the trainer to adequately address such issues he or she must measure, observe, and record the resident's behavior, progress or the lack of it before, during and after each training session. The recording of such data will prove beyond question exactly how much adaptive behavior the resident has gained during each period of training.

Further, evaluation is an ongoing process for the trainer. It helps the trainer by providing him or her with feedback necessary to preserve important data of the resident's performance and reflects the trainers accomplishments and training skills. Likewise, the resident benefits as it identifies the weak points of the training procedures, and assists the trainer and team members to correct them. As a result, it helps the trainer to become more effective in his or her training procedures, and it helps the resident to learn more effectively.

In addition, the critique of the goals and objectives, for all intentions, begins when the program is activated and is continued throughout the period of training. Data is collected, recorded, examined, tracked, and put together into a logical pattern which explains the nature of what the resident is dealing with and relating it to what he or she can do, should do and what can be done. These data collected during the evaluation should raise the following questions. 1) Are the objectives attainable? 2) Are they desirable? and 3) Are they controllable?

Critique means evaluation of the entire process of formulating, writing and implementing the program, goals and objectives. The most important question the evaluation has to answer is were the objectives reached? And if not why not? Also it must raise the question is the program being implemented subjectively or is it being done in a planned, scheduled, and objective manner. Success in completing the objectives cannot be determined without some method of evaluation.

Thus, the evaluation component serves three purposes. First, it permits observation of the residents performance in various steps of training. Second, it makes it possible to evaluate staff performance as they carry out their assigned duties, and three, it supplies the necessary information to allow for important management decisions about the residents treatment program. When these kind of records are being obtained on an ongoing basis, everyone involved in the program has an objective measure of the relative effectiveness of the various components of the treatment plan. Without these three categories of data, it's never clear how the overall program is progressing or how the different components are functioning.

In conclusion, the evaluation process helps the facility in that preserved data allows it to achieve and maintain accreditation to operate as a healthcare provider and the data is available if needed to meet any legal challenges when and if they occur. And more importantly, it allows the activity specialist to measure two extremely important factors: 1) whether the strategies and training procedures are appropriate and effective, and 2) whether the goals and objectives are being met or not. Also, it helps the staff grow, mature, and appreciate the fact that changing behavior requires patience, careful observation, time, hard work, and consistency in their role as caregivers who are responsible for implementing the residents individual therapeutic activity plan. And finally, for the evaluation process to be successful, the activity specialist must have the techniques to measure, analyze, and systematically record observable behavior during training sessions and more specifically during the evaluation process. The following examples are some ways to record behavioral data when doing an evaluation:

James W. Ramage Ph.D.

PROGRAM EVALUATION

FACILITY_____

PROGRAM_____

EVALUATION PROCEDURE_____ TIME _____

PERIOD _____ TO _____

A four step method was used to critique this particular program of service. Examination included assessment of 1) goals, 2) objectives (outcome evaluation), 3) strategies (process evaluation) and 4 methods of evaluation. The purpose of this evaluation was to first insure quality programming and second to collect empirical data that will augment the facility's commitment in meeting the prescribed criteria mandated by Federal and State Regulatory Agencies and appropriate professional community in long-term care facilities. Procedural protocol included assessing, both subjectively and objectively, the following elements of service.

1) Are therapeutic activity programs designed and implemented with specifically written measurable goals and objectives?

Yes _____ No _____ Other _____ Comments_____

_____

2) Do objectives have a start and completion date?

Yes _____ No _____ Other _____ Comments_____

_____

3) Are goals and objectives formulated based upon a diagnostic assessment reflecting team input, continuity of care and addresses the individual needs of each resident?

Yes _____ No _____ Other _____ Comments_____

_____

4) Do formulated activity programming adhere to the principals, standards, policies and procedures of Federal and State Regulatory Agencies and have both financial and emotional support from administration?

Yes _____ No _____ Other _____ Comments_____

_____

5) Does therapeutic activity programming reflect current philosophy of professional recreation community?

Yes _____ No _____ Other _____ Comments_____

_____

6) Are activity programs current, timely and positive?

Yes _____ No _____ Other _____ Comments_____

_____

7) Do formulated strategies reflect a time frame for completion and who, when and how each objective will be addressed to insure completion?

Yes _____ No _____ Other _____ Comments_____

_____

8) Are programs designed to address and promote the residents health, prevent increased disability and impairment and provide habilitation to the resident?

Yes _____ No _____ Other _____ Comments_____

_____

9) Are programs therapeutic in nature, custom designed to address specific physical, mental, emotional and spiritual needs of the resident?

Yes _____ No _____ Other _____ Comments_____

_____

10) Are diagnostic and evaluation procedures evident in assessment of the intellectual, social, spiritual, creative, and physical needs of the resident?

Yes _____ No _____ Other _____ Comments_____

_____

11) Are activities appropriate and meaningful for residents based on their belief system, culture, values, life experiences and interests?

Yes _____ No _____ Other _____ Comments_____

_____

12) Are residents religious, leisure, seasonal, and holiday preferences being addressed?

Yes _____ No _____ Other _____ Comments_____

_____

13) Do activities provide the resident with opportunities for physical, mental and emotional outlets?

Yes _____ No _____ Other _____ Comments_____
_____

14) Do activities promote challenges that instill feelings of usefulness which improves the residents self-worth and self-esteem?

Yes _____ No _____ Other _____ Comments_____
_____

15) Do activities address both short and long term memory span of the resident?

Yes _____ No _____ Other _____ Comments_____
_____

16) Do programs provide the resident with the opportunity to increase/maintain their self-help and practical living skills (ADLS)?

Yes _____ No _____ Other _____ Comments_____
_____

17) Do programs provide resident(s) with outdoor experiences with animals, birds, nature and children?

Yes _____ No _____ Other _____ Comments_____
_____

18) Do programs provide opportunity for resident(s) to participate in both small and large group activities to improve their socialization skills?

Yes _____ No _____ Other _____ Comments_____

19) Are family, spouse, relative and support groups included in the resident's habilitation?

Yes _____ No _____ Other _____ Comments_____

20) Is pastoral counseling included in treatment plans to assist the resident with religious, death and dying issues?

Yes _____ No _____ Other _____ Comments_____

SUMMARY OF FINDINGS, COMMENTS, AND RECOMMENDATIONS.

SIGNATURE OF CONSULTANT

TRAINING PROFICIENCY SCALE

PURPOSE: To evaluate proficiency in using operant conditioning teachniques.

INSTRUCTIONS: For each item rate the trainer on a 2 point scale.

KEY: G = Good   NI = Needs Improvement

TRAINER: RESIDENT:

RATER: _____   DATE: ___

SCHEDULED TIME: TIME OF
                         ___   TRAINING: ___

LOCATION: _____   SKILL: _____

BEHAVIOR	RATING
1) Prepares for training	
2) Uses client's name before command (Obtain client's attention)	
3) Uses verbal prompts correctly	
4) Uses demonstration correctly	
5) Uses gestural prompts correctly	
6) Uses physical prompts correctly	
7) Uses manipulative prompts correctly	
8) Uses reinforcement correctly	
9) Scores data sheet correctly	
10) Uses the proper sequence of prompts	

11) Correctly handles inappropriate behavior of client during training
12) Conducts training as scheduled

COMMENTS:

_____

_____

_____

_____

_____

EVALUATION OF ACTIVITY PROGRAM AND STAFF EFFECTIVENESS
EXAMPLE

AREA	QUESTIONS
1) Program	Is It Appropriate, Timely, Needed?
2) Objectives	Outcome of Training Being Met?
3) Strategies	Training Procedures Working?
4) Atmosphere and Relationships	What Kind? How Close?
5) Member Participation	How Much? How Equal?
6) Goal Understanding and Acceptance	Amount Needed? How Equal?
7) Listening and Information Sharing	How? To Whom?
8) Handling Disagreements and Conflict	How to Handle? Resolution?
9) Decision Making	Who? How?
10) Evaluation of Member Performance	How? By Whom?
11) Expressing Feelings	How? In What Manner?
12) Division of Labor	How? By Whom?
13) Leadership	What Kind? How Appointed?
14) Attention to Process	How? Procedures?

Ratings: 1) Excellent _____
2) Good _____
3) Average _____
4) Fair _____
5) Poor _____

Evaluator _____

Date _____

VIII.   A Review of Doing Evaluation.

Definition: A method of collecting empirical data which provides information about the success of training program.

It insures quality control and accountability.

It provides the trainer an opportunity to begin critiquing program when objectives are activated and promotes continuity throughout each training session.

It tells the trainer whether the strategies for implementing the objectives are working or not and if not, why.

It tells the trainer if the objective is met, can be completed as written, or if instead it should be revised or discontinued.

It affords the trainer the opportunity to assess the objectives to insure that they are

* Measurable
* Observable
* Outcome – Oriented
* Time Limited
* Test Residents Competency
* Positive
* Sequential Developed
* Realistic
* Doable
* Manageable
* Understandable

CHAPTER TEN

INSERVICE TRAINING

Inservice Training conducted in a nursing home facility is often viewed as a necessary evil. This not only holds true for administrative personnel, but also for professional and supportive personnel as well. And as a result, this very vital and important aspect of a nursing home program is often de-emphasized and in many instances sadly neglected. However, if a well-balanced, well-integrated and diversified program of services is being pursued, then a well-planned inservice training program will be implemented. Not only is it a valuable tool in resolving conflicts, friction and discontentment among staff members, but it tends to bolster the morale of employees. And as a result, an inservice training program can instill a sense of security in employees which is vital as insecurity among staff members is difficult to hide from the resident population. It is difficult because residents tend to monitor moods, attitudes, and feelings among employees just as children do with their parents. Hence, one of the goals of an inservice training program is to create a sense of security in the employees.

The basis of any inservice training should be to give the employee a clear and complete understanding of his or her position in the nursing home facility, his or her specific job and the reasons his or her job is necessary. It should also serve to assist him or her in gaining the knowledge and skills necessary to perform his or her job in a satisfactory manner.

In establishing an inservice training program in a nursing home facility, emphasis should first be placed on orientation to the home. A description of the purpose of the home and the reasons for its existence is of major importance. Although a tour of the home along with an introduction to other staff members is necessary, it is of secondary importance to a thorough introduction to the nursing home. Also, if one exists, the employee should be provided with a handbook which should repeat the description of the objectives of the home. It should also give the employee a complete listing of the basis for his or her employment. And in addition, it provides his or her with data pertaining to vacation, sick leave, rules pertaining to conduct, reasons for termination of employment and information regarding time, place and method of distribution of salary.

During the orientation process, a description of the various other employees in the home should be included. Emphasis should be placed on their respective roles in fulfilling the mission of the nursing home facility and its total program of services with direct reference to the roles of the various employees. In this way, when a worker reaches this assignment, he or she will understand how his or her department fit into the total program of services, and how both relate to other departments and employees in the home. Also the use of various organizational charts can be an effective method of orienting the employee.

Also, orientation should include a good job description for each position in the home. This is important because a job description is the basis for the employees orientation to his or her specific function. And in it the employee should find a clearly defined description of his or her duties, responsibilities, the method for accounting to his or her superiors for meeting responsibilities which he or she is assigned, as well as an indication of what he or she may expect in the way of additional duties and responsibilities. And, in addition, if it is required, a job description might be included to inform him or her how he or she is expected to do his or her job, and standards which may be applied to his or her performance. Also, matters regarding dress and personal appearance might be included, as well as a description of the conduct which will be demanded of him or her in his or her relationships and dealings with his superiors, co-workers, residents and visitors to the home. The job description, if a detailed description is given, should give the employees all the basic rules of his or her job. A good job description is often beneficial as it allows the employee to refer to it should he or she have a particular question which has not been made clear when the same item was being described to him or her during the orientation process to his or her job.

Thus, the foundation upon which an administrator can build an effective and productive inservice training program is orientation. Without a complete and comprehensive orientation, an inservice training program has far less meaning and can be much more difficult to implement.

It is important for the individual responsible for inservice training to be aware that in each job the employee will have to learn some basic skills. Some employees will come to their job with prior education or training in the assignments which they are given. Others will have to be trained from the start. Regardless of the situation, it should be the duty of each supervisor to assure him or herself that the employee is given complete information regarding the methods to be used in his specific job in the home. Obviously, not all tasks are carried out in the same manner in each nursing home, even on the professional level; therefore, training must be given immediately to each employee in the systems and techniques used in this new position. The reasons for this are to assure that there is uniformity in quality of performance and to permit administrative evaluation of the work done by the employee at a later date.

When possible, a written description of the job skills and techniques should be available to each employee; however, when this is not available, the department in which he or she works should have a complete procedure manual where matters of this type are covered. This is especially important in the nursing department. Also, if the home is to be efficiently run, detailed procedure manuals should be made readily available in at least the housekeeping and dietary departments.

Another objective of an inservice training program is to increase employees' skills as these skills are described in the manuals. And the manuals should come under continuous review as to avoid having them become out of date or ineffective because they do not reflect new techniques, new product usage, and new programs of service.

Although the administrator is not usually a professional at programming inservice training in the nursing home, it is important that his or her administrative manual which includes all other manuals must also be kept as current as possible. Without a current and complete administrative manual, relationships between responsible department heads and administration will prove difficult and much of the valuable time of the administrator will be spent in handling details which might be better handled by those who report to him or her.

It is not unusual to find administrators who consider their inservice training program complete at the point the employee has received the basic orientation training for his or her job. They assume that an adequate orientation to the home and to the job, along with training and skills required to accomplish the job, is significant and is the full extent of a proper inservice training program. This, of course, is not true. At this point the job is only half done. The true purpose of a complete inservice training program is to train and thereby retrain experienced employees. The objective is to assist the employee to develop in his or her job, to increase the satisfaction he or she gets from doing his or her job, to further his or her understanding of the mission of the home and his or her roles in accomplishing that mission and to increase his or her security by permitting him or her to measure his performance against the standards established for him or her. The result of post-orientation inservice training programs will be improved in the worker's thinking, behavior, skills and interpersonal relationships and habits of work. And, finally, a complete inservice training program will introduce an exchange of ideas on how the job can be better done and how to bring about the improvements through the introduction of change.

The changing of programs, procedures, requirements and techniques are a common occurrence in the nursing home which is active. They are indications of the rapid increase in knowledge regarding the care of the chronically ill as well as the results of the ever tightening relationship between the dynamic science of medicine and the modern nursing home facility.

Change is always threatening to employees because it introduces new demands and skills. The employee's security is threatened by change and he or she will resist it because of fear of unknown demands or skills. If the home is to progress, however, it must always improve and if it is constantly changing, there is an ever present need to retrain each employee so he or she will fully understand the change and its impact on the job and the home. It is always desirable when a major change in operation occurs, for it to be preceded by complete orientation and training. In this way, the employee will have the advantage of knowing about the change prior to its being made, and of having the security of knowing how to do his job properly at the time of change. This will tend to build an increasingly loyal and skilled staff for the nursing home.

And, the inservice training program must take into account yet another problem. This is the problem created by the fact that most of the care given to the resident is given by the staff members with the least amount of formal education or training. There is a continuous need for intensive training of these individuals who relate to residents on an individual basis. There are no two human beings alike, therefore, there is no such thing as a correct method of handling all patients in all situations. With the increase in the incidence of mental and emotional problems in the nursing home, there is a demand for initiative, intelligence, tact, and a higher degree of understanding in giving resident care. These can be acquired only after a prolonged period of training and observation. The aides and orderlies and other supportive personnel must have continuous and intensive inservice training programs in order that they may learn how they can improve their skills and why the residents react as they do. Without such training and guidance, the staff members will develop habits and procedures with residents which may be of assistance to some and of great hindrance to others.

In summary, all nursing home personnel should have the opportunity, in a learning situation, to discuss the handling of residents, problems in relating to residents, and the needs of residents which may be going unfulfilled. The inservice training sessions should be conducted by a person of unquestionable understanding and competence otherwise the instructor may fail in his or her mission of supervising the care of the resident by giving improper advice or misinformation. The continual inservice training of nursing home personnel assigned to and working with residents suffering from dementia is a complex and difficult matter important enough to demand attention to the administrator and financial resources of the nursing home facility.

CHAPTER ELEVEN

ADDRESSING MALADAPTIVE BEHAVIORS

There are times when a noticeable change in a resident's behavior occurs – a depressed mood, episodes of crying, periods of irritability, and restlessness. These behaviors are characterized by withdrawal from social events, recreational activities, interaction with staff, peers and immediate family members alike. Also residents often experience a loss of appetite, have conflicts with his or her caretakers, and they are often combative during ADLs. The following activities are suggested as a means of reducing these behaviors which are symptomatic of depression, anxiety, acting out, combative or conflict. They are: Sensory Soothers Touch: (Being near staff, holding hands with staff while walking), Sensory Soothers Taste: (Chewing ice, eating ice pops, milk shakes), Hygiene Activities (cleaning self, combing hair, washing hands), Manipulative (playing with musical instruments: bells, drums, triangles, autoharp), Motor activities (games involving throwing, range of motion activities: walking).

When participating in these activities, there is less conflict with others, less restlessness and more interaction with staff. While doing these activities, the following is recommended.

1) Praise: When praising the resident, always emphasize the accomplishment, the participation in a "hard activity", and not focus on the performance or the 'looks' of the program. Additionally, since communication can be a barrier, use hand gestures (wave, signal, point), facial expressions (smile, laugh), and Haptics (therapeutic touch: a pat on the back, stroking, hugs, and holding arm) to praise the resident. A simple handshake or clapping in appreciation, or stroking his or her back or hair gently are easy and acceptable ways to communicate praise to the resident.

2) Movement Activities: Daily exercise and leisure groups that emphasize motor activity (using muscles, range of motion activities such as throwing or kicking activities) as a way to relax. Daily exercise and leisure activities that includes a range of motion activities, stretching, muscle building or walking with staff is highly recommended. This is more successful as an individual activity. To assist the resident, have a staff member demonstrate each step of the exercise, and have him or her seated to be able to see the staff member.

3) Sensory Soothers – Taste & Touch: This is a very simple relaxation activity that can be used when a resident is experiencing symptoms (combativeness, restlessness, facial grimacing). When symptoms occur offer the resident something to eat or drink. When offering these foods consider those that he or she usually enjoys, such as milk shakes, ice cream, sherbet, soft ice, or ice pops. When the resident is enjoying these foods, he or she is usually calmer, more relaxed and cooperative. It is also recommended that staff utilize Haptics: therapeutic touch.

This intervention is simple to use. Simply allow the resident to hold a staff member's hand while walking and during ADLs or pat him or her on the back or gesture for a hug. Additionally, avoid pulling away from the resident when he or she attempts to hold. Avoid sudden movements when using these techniques. When provided with sensory soothers the resident is less restless, and less likely to be combative. For example: If the resident is becoming irritable with staff during grooming or ADLs just stop and offer a milk shake, a drink or some soft ice to chew on, and when he or she is done continue with the training activities.

Or,

If the resident is becoming restless and walking around the nursing home and disrupting others have a staff member hold the resident's hand and walk with him or her. The resident will often calm down, and be less restless during the process.

4) Movement Activities: This is a very successful technique that involves simply getting the resident to move and use some of his or her muscles. This could be simple exercises, throwing a ball, playing tug of war with a towel, or lifting his or her legs up and down. Also, walking with assistance works well. If any symptoms or problems are noted, have a staff member approach the resident and extend their hand and then have staff walk with him or her for 10 or 15 minutes or for as long as they can tolerate. When resident does this, it helps him or her to relax, and often calms him or her down. It is recommended that walking with the resident and allowing him or her to hold a staff members hand become a routine daily exercise.

When a resident(s) experiences episodes of disorientation, and restlessness and combative behaviors. The following is suggested:

1) Establish a routine that is flexible. This sounds confusing, but have a daily routine, including time for waking up, bathing, breakfast, morning stretching, lunch, and an afternoon leisure activity, dinner, and an evening exercise group. The routine should have some flexibility for days in which the resident does not want to do certain things, and remember to give him or her choices and not challenges in his or her activities, however, limit choices to 2 or 3 options.

2) Calendar: Have a large easy to read calendar in the residents room that includes day, month, year and location. Additionally, mark off the days that have passed. When choosing a calendar, the simpler is the better. Make every effort to avoid elaborate calendars that may be confusing. If possible, have decorations that indicate holidays, and season.

3) Grin! Smile! Laugh!: There are times when residents working with his or her task becomes frustrated. One simple intervention is to just grin, smile or laugh. When the resident notices you smiling they smile, mimicing or mirroring the staff and his or her mood will generally improve. This however, can also work the reverse in that if you are tense or have a frustrated look on your face the resident mirrors this and becomes more frustrated. One must always be cautious of the emotions being portrayed as the resident may mirror negative expressions.

4) Utilize Personal Hygiene to relax the resident when he or she is combative, confused or restless. Many times normal relaxation activities fail to help to relax the resident. When these techniques fail, the

resident should be encouraged to do his or her own self care, such as washing his or her hands, combing his or her hair, or being assisted with changing clothes, or nail care to become more relaxed. For example, if the resident is becoming restless, and disturbing other people and relaxing activities have not worked, approach him or her and ask the resident the following questions using gestures and signals to establish communication.

"Mr. Doe... It's getting close to dinner time do you want to go and wash your hands and change clothes?" Point at his hands and shirt and smile.

Or,

"Would you like to go and comb your hair and get your nails cut to get ready for the next activity?" Point to his hair and make combing motions and smile.

By approaching the resident with these familiar activities he is able to feel better about their situations and can be redirected into a soothing activity.

5) Use the residents memory deficits to his or her advantage. If the resident becomes uncooperative or unwilling to do activities like grooming, dressing, or exercise allow her or him to be excused from the scheduled activity. However, in about 10 or 15 minutes try again, as the resident has probably forgotten about the reason why he or she did not want to participate. If he or she does not want to exercise or participate in an activity, stop trying to reschedule it for later. If he or she becomes confused about what is going on simply re-introduce yourself with name

and handshake and start over with telling him or her the date, time, and location.

6) Simple is better: ADLs are more successful when each step and aspect of the activity is simplified. To do this, simplify the room and bathing, grooming equipment. Use a plain room with few distractions. Use solid colored clothes, and towels, and close doors and close curtains over windows. Have the room quiet and a comfortable temperature. Start slowly and assist him or her at each step letting her know what he or she is doing and why. Instead of giving him or her complicated commands break them down into small simple 1 – step parts. For Example: Instead of saying, "Mr. Doe ...come over to the table and sit down".

Say to him:

"Hi, Mr. Doe ... Shake my hand ... Put your hand here (gesture to your hand), Stand ... Look up ... Follow me ... Take a step ... Right... Left ... Right ... Left ... Look up ... Now put your hand here (gesture to the table)...Now put your hand here (gesture to the chair), Let go of my hand (gesture to his hand), Put your hand here (gesture to the chair), Then (gesture with hand) and say, 'sit' ... (pat the chair with your hand)".

Often during ADLs: grooming, dressing, bathing, and toileting the resident becomes restless. When he or she attempts to leave before the activity is complete, u se redirection, and give simple One Step Instructions to help him or her complete the activity. Remember to point at objects (clothes, the toilet, soap, running water, or towels) and speak loudly in a kind, firm low toned voice. Additionally, keep an affectionate facial expression. By using these interventions bathing and other daily activities will be more successful, and the resident will exhibit fewer symptoms of inappropriate behavior.

7) Choices Not Challenges: Remember when providing care for resident(s) provide him or her with choices and not challenge, to ensure feelings of independence. For Example: if you are trying to help the resident to get dressed avoid saying things that might sound like challenges or commands, such as: "You need to put on your shirt... You have to wear a pair of shoes... You need to do your exercises now... It's time to eat, eat now."

When possible avoid such challenges and give the resident choices to allow feelings of independence. Statements like these allow the resident choices and fewer challenges: While making the statements hold up the clothing items and let the resident point to the one he or she wants to wear. During meals let the resident point to the foods he or she wants to eat first. By stating choices and allowing the resident to point and choose he or she exhibits less of their symptoms.

"Mr. Doe, which shirt would you like to wear today... red or blue? Would you like to wear your white or brown shoes today? Would you like to eat a snack now or later? Would you like to eat the chicken or dessert first? Would you like to exercise or rest here in your chair?"

By giving the resident choices in their daily activities you will avoid challenges and he or she will exhibit more appropriate behavior and have a better quality of life. When considering activities to assist with these behaviors, the following should be entertained:

Arts and crafts such as working with repetition tasks (painting activities, decorating),

Reminiscing groups (sharing stories, talking about antiques),

Individual activities (looking through magazines, reading from the Bible),

Leisure activities (Bingo, card games: rook, throwing games, competitive games),

Motor activities (kicking and throwing games, range of motion activities).

When the resident does these activities he or she is not as worried or preoccupied, has less conflict with others, and improved self esteem. While doing these activities the following is suggested:

Getting resident to large and small group sessions.

1) Encouragement and Education: Encourage the resident to attend each group and inform group members about how the group can help him or her better, and let them know how it will benefit him or her. For example, if there is a group activity scheduled state to the resident:

"Good morning, there is an exercise activity in the day room, it will be a good opportunity to stretch and make your legs stronger, and a good chance for you to be with other people". Also emphasize the benefits of the group:

"A game of bingo is beginning in the day room, it would be a good opportunity to exercise your mind and at the same time have some fun."

2) Leisure Activities: Leisure based (games with prizes) or craft based (something the resident can make for him or herself or a family mem-

ber). Be sure to invite resident to group activities that include prizes or crafts and educate him or her about what he or she can "win" in the group or "make".

3) Current Events/Magazines: Many residents enjoy reading and discussing the local news with staff and residents. A good activity would be to invite him or her and other residents with staff and have them take turns reading short articles from the paper and talk about their opinions. Additionally, if he or she enjoys looking at picture magazines that are based on leisure, food or travel, or any magazine with big pictures in it keeps the residents attention and they enjoy looking through them. It is recommended that a nice supply of magazines be made available for them. Many also enjoy making scrapbooks out of the pictures they like. Simply allow the resident to tear out pictures and using glue or tape compile the pictures on construction paper to make a collage or scrapbooks. Scrapbook themes can be favorite foods, houses, flowers, recipes, cars, pets...etc. Additionally utilize the following interventions when the resident attends a group or activity:

1) Praise: Praise the resident, always emphasizing his/her accomplishments, and degree of participation.

2) Physical Exercise: Offer daily exercise and leisure groups that emphasize motor activity (using muscles, range of motion activities) as a way to relax and alleviate anxiety (worry). It is recommended that the resident be offered daily exercise and leisure activities that includes range of motion activities, stretching, and muscle building. Offering the exercise in a group is best as the resident is given the opportunity

to participate in exercises. To assist the resident, have a staff member demonstrate each step of the exercise, and have him or her seated to be able to see the staff member.

3) Relaxation: While working on these activities the resident often becomes frustrated and makes more mistakes and eventually attempts to quit doing the task. Often times he or she becomes preoccupied about somatic complaints, such as a headache or 'sinus problems'. By having the resident do simple Deep Breathing exercises, or do some steps of progressive muscle relaxation he or she can avoid getting irritable or frustrated about his or her situation or feeling bad about their abilities. If complaints of sinus or headache continue, seek medical consultation. Often times these physical complaints and worries are symptoms of the resident's illness and you should encourage him or her to relax first, and then evaluate the issues. Intervening or somatization symptoms can be difficult at times, if you require assistance contact professional in charge for further instructions.

4) Self – Concept: Participating in these activities helps to build more confidence and self-esteem. Specifically, doing daily exercise or simple crafts will give the resident the confidence he or she needs to continue doing things that make them happy. While working on these projects praise the resident for his or her accomplishments.

5) Past Success: One very simple intervention that helps to get the resident to engage or attend is to remind him or her of the past successes he or she has had in similar activities. For example, if the resident is reluctant to attend a craft group, say:

"Mr. Doe, I hear that you are not interested in doing the crafts, but the last time you worked on your project you had a really good time, and you were proud of what you did. Let's go work on this project and have a good time".

Or, if he is reluctant to come to an exercise group you could say:

"I understand that you don't feel like exercising today, the last time you came to the exercise group you had a good time and you were smiling and having fun. Let's go try to exercise again."

6) Concentration Skills: Doing these types of activities may seem simple, but they are designed to help the resident with building and maintaining his or her concentration level. Remember to focus on the enjoyment, and benefits of the task versus the overall usefulness of the item you are making.

7) Reminiscing Activities: The residents often enjoy doing several reminiscing activities. During these group activities, group members are encouraged to share stories from the past that are amusing, interesting, or inspiring. Often times these discussions are started by sharing a story from a book or a magazine. Two very good sources used by many facilities for starting a reminiscing group are Reminisce Magazine, Good Old Days Magazine, or Country.

8) Positive Self – Talk: There are times when the resident is trying to work on a project or while doing an activity that they begin to say and think less of him or herself. They will talk negatively about themselves (saying 'I can't hear well enough', 'Take me to my room', 'I can't do that,

it's too hard') or the thing they are working on (being overly critical, saying 'it's no good').

Gently point this out to the resident that he or she is using Negative Self-Talk, and how that it is unhealthy to dwell on the negatives. Then have the resident to relax and start using positive thinking skills. For example:

If he or she is saying: "Oh, I keep on making mistakes, I can't do the project any more"; Have the resident STOP, and relax by taking several Deep Breaths and have him or her say "I am making some mistakes, BUT I can take a break and I can try it again"; OR, if they are saying: "My sinuses are acting up too much I can't breathe, take me to bed, I want to rest, I can't do this anymore, I am going to quit..."

Have the resident to STOP, and relax by clinching and relaxing his or her hands (making tight fists) and have him or her say:

"I am not as healthy as I used to be, BUT I can take a break and then I can work on it later without having to quit".

Those residents exhibiting excessive worry, preoccupations with somatic complaints, acting out behaviors, conflict with staff and residents can benefit from the following strategies. Relaxation: Practiced several different types of relaxation exercises such as: deep breathing, daily exercise, some steps of progressive muscle relaxation.

Have the resident practice each of these and be able to use them when prompted by staff member. When the resident is prompted by staff to use them, a significant decrease in the resident's symptoms is usually observed.

Listed below are a few tips on how to do the relaxing activities to help the resident to deal with anxiety and reduce preoccupations.

1) Routine: Build a daily routine, that includes doing one relaxation exercise during the daytime to help relax, a good time is 1:30 P.M. and in the evening times.

2) Examples: At times these activities are hard to do, and the resident does well when he or she is able to follow along with someone, so perform the activity yourself and have him or her mimic you while you are doing each step of the activity.

3) Variety: Change up the routine and try different relaxation techniques.

4) Comfortable and quiet: Try to utilize a room that is comfortable and quiet.

5) Dim the Lights: This simple step makes the relaxation activity beneficial.

6) Redirection and Distraction: If the resident is acting out or becoming irritated with others or talking about something that is making them mad (delusional thoughts) or frustrated, attempts to redirect the conversation by distracting him or her either to talk about another topic (reminiscing) or into a simple relaxation activity (deep breathing, muscle relaxation).

7) Use as needed. If the resident is showing symptoms (disorientation, preoccupation, excessive worry, irritability, acting out behaviors

or conflicts) have him or her to do one of the relaxation exercises. For example: If you notice that the resident is becoming disoriented or irritable, say to him or her.

"I know you are frustrated being here. Let's try to relax by taking three slow deep breaths, follow along with me and I will help you relax... then we can talk about what is troubling you"...

Then have resident practice the deep breathing relaxation routine and talk about his or her feelings. Or

If he or she is preoccupied about things, say:

"Mr. Doe, I know you are having some troubles with your thinking, and it worries you a lot. Lets try to relax. Follow along with me, we can relax and then see what is wrong. Okay?" Then have him practice some of the progressive muscle relaxation routines to relax. Encourage him to do simple craft activities like working in a coloring book.

8) Use of Medications: As a last resort, if the resident is still unable to relax by doing a relaxation activity, consult medical staff to offer education about medications that are prescribed to assist with the symptoms. Following the education process, remind the resident that it is okay to take medicine to help with his or her illness.

And finally, inappropriate sexual behaviors, in the elderly and more specifically among those residents suffering from dementia especially those residing in long term care facilities remain the most sensitive and controversial issues in the health care industry. This is true largely on the part of the resident, because he or she with dementing illnesses Experiences changes in their cognition and judgment. Therefore, their expression of Sexuality often results in inappropriate sexual behaviors that are unacceptable at home or community and are challenging to manage in the environment of a health care facility. This is true also on the part of family members in that values, morays, and attitudes which continue to linger around sexuality in society. Then, too, the health care provider is often ill trained in the psychology of dealing with sexuality and associated problems with the resident and their families in long term care facilities.

Psychology teaches that all human beings need to be held, caressed and touched first as an infant and this need continues throughout life. This is especially true for the elderly resident suffering from Alzheimer's disease. However, such behavior should be exhibited appropriately in appropriate places, times and conditions. When such behavior is exhibited inappropriately in appropriate places, at inappropriate times and under inappropriate conditions, it results in behavior which family members, spouse, significant others, or caregivers find embarrassing, threatening and disturbing. Such behavior sooner or later, usually sooner, results in placement in a long term care facility. Such inappropriate sexual behaviors consists of the following:

º Social dysfunction/uninhibited sexual behavior in the home or community

º Inappropriate sexual remarks

º Exposing him or herself

º Masturbating in public

º Voroism

º Propositioning others for sex

º Grabbing or fondling others

º Flirting or making unwanted sexual advances towards members of the opposite sex

º Attempting to dress or undress at inappropriate times and places performing or soliciting oral sex

º Making sexual advances toward strangers who resembles a former spouse or companion

º Making unwanted sexual advances toward children and teenagers

º Having frequent episodes of unreasonable jealous and suspicious behavior, accusing spouse of unfaithfulness and unfounded illicit sexual behavior.

The following examples of the activities are some which are suggested as a means of reducing these behaviors. They are as follows:

º Listen to and respond carefully to threats and accusations and redirect resident to another activity reassuring him or her with motor activities (walking exercises) and sensory soothers (touching, hugging, stroking, rubbing).

º Assess for a reason for the behavior – he or she may be searching for the bathroom, taking off his or her clothes getting ready for bed or have a medical problem such as a urinary tract infection. Motor movement such as walking exercises, redirection, hygiene and motor activities reduce his or her anxiety.

º Approach resident with patience and gentleness: remind with calm voice that such sexual behavior is inappropriate. Redirect resident to private place and avoid getting angry or making jokes out of behavior. Movement activities, walking exercises, praise, sensory soothers, touch, pat, hug can help the resident reduce his or her acting out.

° Patiently adjust or change clothing. This cannot be a restraint but put the residents pants or dress on backwards or provide him or her with pull-on trousers without buttons or zipper. Motor activities, throwing games, range of motion activities, walking exercises are helpful in helping the resident calm his or her behavior.

° Increase level of emotional and physical contact to calm. Movement activities – walking exercises, sensory soothers: touch, stroking, patting, hugging, and rubbing, along with reassurance through gentle touching, soft, loving communication, assist in reducing the residents irritability and restlessness.

° Adjust to changes in sexual desire of spouses, sleeping apart, demanding attitude, or because of jealous or irrational behavior. Movement activities, walking exercises, sensory soothers, being near staff, holding hands with staff while walking, physical exercise: using muscles, range of motion, stretching, concentration skills such as focusing games are helpful in assisting the resident with depression, periods of irritability, restlessness, combative behavior and conflicts.

Seek professional help to cope with sexual issues. As program of treatment begins, activities can be prescribed which compliment and augment the treatment process such as sensory soothers, taste to reward appropriate and desired response, praise to emphasize accomplishment, encouragement/education exercises to assist the resident understand sexual issues.

However, before any activity is implemented the recreator should make sure that he or she has an activity, or is capable of designing one which first addresses the residents need(s), and second will do so in a therapeutic manner. And once written the activity should be thoroughly critiqued. This is necessary to make sure that the prescribed activity is therapeutic by reflecting a specific, goal – directed therapy, based upon a working diagnostic assessment to insure that it is attainable, desirable, and controllable. The following examples reflect several behaviors frequently exhibited by residents and activities prescribed to address them in several facilities providing special care to residents suffering from dementia.

THERAPEUTIC ACTIVITY

Behavior Targeted: Wandering.

Behavior Defined: Pacing or roaming about facility for no rational reason.

Activity Prescribed: Reality orientation/small group activities.

Goal: To reduce wandering.

Objective: Within three (3) months resident will reduce his/her wandering to three (3) episodes or less per shift with verbal prompting from the trainer.

Steps:

1) Always approach resident in a calm and patient manner and speak in a calm voice.
2) Re-orientate resident to his/her room.
3) Orientate resident to facility.
4) Engage resident in small group activities (movement activities).
5) Monitor resident's location with visual checks every hour.
6) Place items with which the resident is familiar on door and his/her room.

7) Attempt to find out for what the resident is searching or looking.

8) When found wandering escort him/her back to his/her room and orientate to location and familiar item near or in his/her room.

9) Report any physical symptoms to medical staff.

THERAPEUTIC ACTIVITY

Behavior Targeted: Adjustment/Separation Anxieties.

Behavior Defined: Repetitive statements of unhappiness, of wanting to go home.

Activity Prescribed: Reality therapy/movement activities/ sensory soothers.

Goal: To improve social skills.

Objective: Within three (3) months the resident will reduce his or her episodes of physical and verbal resistance to nursing home environment to three (3) or less incidents per week with verbal prompts by the trainer.

Steps:

1) Approach resident calmly and unhurriedly. Speak in a kind and calm voice.

2) Assist resident to begin to participate in dining program in dining room.

3) Assist resident to begin to participate in movement activities.

4) Assist resident with socialization with roommate and other residents.

5) Assist with socialization with room visits for reality therapy.

6) Encourage family to visit in room and facility.

7) Encourage community outings (dining, hair appointments).

8) Reinforce with praise for any and all appropriate behavior.

9) Report any medical symptoms to medical staff.

THERAPEUTIC ACTIVITY

Behavior Targeted: Paranoia, Delusions, Hallucinations.

Behavior Defined: Suspiciousness, distrustfulness, inappropriate statements, seeing and hearing things and voices that aren't present.

Activity Prescribed: A combination of reality orientation/movement activity/sensory soothers.

Goal: To reduce conversations with imaginary people.

Objective: Within three (3) months the resident will reduce episodes of talking to imaginary people to three (3) per week by participating in reality orientation, movement and sensory soother activities when verbally prompted by the trainer.

Steps:

1) Approach the resident in a calm and patient manner. Speak in a kind and calm voice.
2) Post resident's picture and name on door to room. Also pictures of family, along with familiar things from his/her home along with a large calendar.
3) Listen and observe carefully and attentively.

4) Ignore all references to imaginary people.

5) Attempt to make resident validate and refocus from negative to positive things.

6) Assist resident in determining what is real from unreal.

7) Reassure the resident of his/her safety when upset.

8) Inservice the staff, caretakers, and family to relate to resident in same manner.

9) Report any physical symptoms to medical personnel.

THERAPEUTIC ACTIVITY

Behavior Targeted: Excessive worry and anxiety.

Behavior Defined: Shaking, pacing, continuous movement, frequent use of call light, demanding attention, repetitive verbal statements and nervousness.

Prescribed Activity: Movement Activities/Sensory Soothers.

Goal: To reduce worry and anxiety.

Objective: Within three (3) months resident will reduce episodes of worrying and anxiety to ten (10) minutes per week by walking a distance of twenty (20) feet twice a day when physically prompted to do so by trainer without stopping for rest on five (5) consecutive days.

Steps:

1) Approach resident in a calm, firm, and patient manner – speaking in a kind but firm voice.

2) Listen attentively and attempt to resolve or discuss area which is upsetting to resident.

3) Attempt to define reason or cause for worry and anxiety.

4) In room visitation at least three (3) times a week for socialization activities.

5) Assist resident to define interest and concerns.

6) Reassure resident when episode of excess worry or anxiety occurs.

7) When resident is upset take on walk and reinforce positive behavior with praise.

8) Report any physical symptoms to medical personnel.

THERAPEUTIC ACTIVITY

Behavior Targeted: Depression.

Behavior Defined: A sudden change in behavior going from a happy state to a sad or angry one for no apparent reason, withdrawal from social events and activities, periods of laughing or crying for no obvious reason, a change in eating and sleeping habits.

Activity Prescribed: Small group, movement and sensory soother activities.

Goal: To reduce depression.

Objective: Within three (3) months the resident will have less than three (3) episodes per week of laughing and crying for no apparent reason for two consecutive weeks.

Steps:

1) Approach resident in a kind, firm and patient manner.
2) Listen attentively and attempt to define or resolve area which is upsetting.
3) Reassure resident when he or she is upset.

4) In room visits to reassure and motivate resident to leave room to attend activities, especially dining.

5) Assist resident in altering his or her environment, involve in movement activities, sensory soothers, and small group activities.

6) Report any medical symptoms to medical personnel.

James W. Ramage Ph.D.

THERAPEUTIC ACTIVITY

Behavior Targeted: Combative behavior.

Behavior Defined: Striking, hitting, slapping, spitting, kicking.

Activity Prescribed: Movement activities, sensory soothers, relaxation exercises.

Goal: To reduce hitting.

Objective: Within three (3) months resident will have three (3) or less episodes of hitting per week by participating in relaxation exercises, and brisk walks following each episode of hitting to calm, with physical prompts from trainer on five (5) consecutive days.

Steps:

1) Approach resident in a calm and patient manner. Speak in a kind, but firm voice. Assume authoritative stance.
2) Listen attentively.
3) Explain all procedures and reason to resident before performing.
4) Attempt to refocus negative behavior to something positive when resident is upset and exhibiting abusive behavior.
5) Redirect away from group to take deep breathing exercises to calm.

186

6) Assist resident to help staff in mutual problem solving of abusive causing stimuli.

7) Assist resident in participating in movement activity (walking).

8) Assist resident in discussing his or her interests and concerns.

9) Involve family in community outings.

10) Report any physical symptoms to medical staff.

THERAPEUTIC ACTIVITY

Behavior Targeted: Confusion.

Behavior Defined: Unaware of time, place, people, events, getting lost, demonstrates fearful behavior.

Activity Prescribed: Reality orientation.

Goal: Improve cognitive skills.

Objective: The resident will remember his or her room by seeing familiar objects and photographs of family members on or near door on five (5) of seven (7) days per week independently by _____ _____ (date).

Steps:

1) Always approach resident calmly and in an unhurried manner.

2) Speak in a calm non-threatening, reassuring voice.

3) Explain all procedures and reasons before performing.

4) Listen attentively, maintain non-threatening facial expressions.

5) Involve in enjoyable cognitive challenging activities which orient to reality – reward with praise for all positive behavior.

6) Encourage family and close relatives to visit.

7) Post photos and mementos on door and in room.

8) All interaction with resident should be pleasant and non-threatening to reassure the resident during episodes of confusion.

9) Place his or her name on outside of room; keep current calendar in his or her room.

10) Involve in small group sessions; encourage reminiscing.

11) Assist in emergencies.

12) Verbal prompts to assist resident with orientation.

THERAPEUTIC ACTIVITY

Behavior Targeted: Anger.

Behavior Defined: Verbal expressions of anger, throwing things, striking out, cursing, withdrawal from social events, refusing to participate in activities, refusing to come out of his or her room, refusing to eat and rejection of care or medical treatments.

Activity Prescribed: Movement activities/ relaxation exercises.

Goal: Reduce anger.

Objective: Resident will have less than three (3) episodes of throwing things on five (5) of seven (7) days per week with verbal prompts from trainer by _____ (date).

Steps:

1) Approach resident in calm and in an unhurried manner.
2) Speak to resident in calm, kind but firm voice.
3) Listen to resident in an attentive manner.
4) Redirect residents negative behavior to something positive when the resident is exhibiting abusive behavior.
5) When he/she is demonstrating abusive outbursts, calmly ask resident to take some deep breaths and to calm down.

6) Encourage and assist the resident to help staff in mutual problem solving of abusive causing stimuli.

7) Redirect resident away from group and participate in walking and relaxation exercises.

8) Encourage resident to discuss interests and concerns.

9) Involve family in resident's habilitation.

THERAPEUTIC ACTIVITY

Behavior Targeted: Conflicts.

Behavior Defined: Frequent complaints and arguments with peers and staff members, makes up untrue stories about other residents or caregivers.

Activity (s) Prescribed: Movement activities/ relaxation exercises.

Goal: Reduce conflicts.

Objective: The resident will make less than three (3) complaints per week about caregivers by _____ (date).

Steps:

1) Visit the resident frequently to see if he or she needs anything.

2) Always approach resident in calm and unhurried manner.

3) Speak in a kind but firm manner.

4) Listen to resident attentively for complaints.

5) When resident is exhibiting inappropriate behavior attempt to refocus negative behavior to something positive.

6) Encourage and assist the resident to help staff in mutual problem solving of conflicts causing stimuli.

7) Attempt to investigate and resolve complaints.

8) Redirect away from group and engage resident in movement activities (walking) and relaxation (deep breathing) exercises.

9) Encourage resident to discuss his or her interests and concerns.

10) Change residents caregiver or roommate if it is determined that it may resolve problems.

11) Involve family in resident's care.

THERAPEUTIC ACTIVITY

Behavior Targeted: Mood Disorder.

Behavior Defined: Signs or symptoms of resident going from happy to sad to anger quickly for no apparent reason.

Activity Prescribed: Movement activities (walking), sensory soothers, relaxation exercises (deep breathing), (taste and touch).

Goal: To reduce mood swings.

Objective: The resident will have less than three (3) episodes per week of laughing and crying for no apparent reason by _____
_____ (date).

Steps:

1) When resident is exhibiting episodes of laughing and crying and in general exhibiting inappropriate behavior(s), the staff will attempt to alter the resident's environment by redirecting to quite area away from group.
2) Involve in movement activities (walking exercises).
3) Relaxation exercises (deep breathing exercises, taste and touch).
4) Reassure resident when he or she is observed exhibiting inappropriate laughing or crying.

5) Attempt to evaluate cause for residents inappropriate laughing or crying.

6) Listen attentively and attempt to discuss why the resident is upset.

THERAPEUTIC ACTIVITY

Behavior targeted: Insomnia.

Behavior Defined: Resident seems nervous, sleeps most of the day, makes statements that they didn't sleep, staying in their rooms, or are ill tempered.

Activity Prescribed: Movement activities (throwing – pitching games, range of motion activities and walking exercises).

Goal: To improve sleep.

Objective: Within three months, the resident will sleep six (6) to eight (8) hours per night on at least five (5) or seven (7) days each week.

Steps:

1) Always approach resident in calm and relaxed manner.
2) Speak to resident with kind but firm voice.
3) Listen attentively.
4) Attempt to define what is the cause of inability to sleep.
5) Encourage – assist the resident to stay up during the day to enable him or her to sleep at night.
6) Monitor causes for insomnia – caffeine, over stimulation, fear, death and dying issues, adjustment and separation anxieties.

7) Encourage – insist that resident actively participate in such activities as walking, hygiene activities (cleaning self, grooming), manipulatives (playing musical instruments such as bells, drums, triangles, etc.), motor activities (throwing – pitching games, range of motion activities).

CHAPTER TWELVE

WRITING BEHAVIOR MANAGEMENT PLANS

This chapter addresses the management of disruptive and inappropriate behavior. More specifically, it focuses on managing aggressive behavior in the elderly suffering from Alzheimer's Disease and doing it in the most humane and least intrusive manner possible. When addressing aggressive and disruptive behavior it is generally accepted that one is referring to an aggressive act or acts towards one's self or towards another individual in his or her presence. These aggressive acts are characterized by self-destructive, bizarre and stereotyped behavior, outbursts of anger, negativism and in general, rebelliousness and a refusal to comply and cooperate. It provides an overview of the delivery of behavioral programming provided for those residents suffering from dementia who exhibit acts of disruptive behavior often enough and severe enough to require an individualized behavior management plan.

A behavior management plan should never be taken lightly nor should they be written routinely. They should be written in two (2) basic forms: 1) to address a specific behavior, in a specific setting for a specific individual and 2) to address a specific behavior problem for a specific individual. And then, it should only be written following a comprehensive assessment (including behavioral, medical, psychiatric, social, religious and recreational) and analysis (including a behavioral or functional analysis) which is extremely important and should include the following:

1) Definition of the behavior being targeted;

2) A scatter plot of targeted behaviors during the past thirty (30) days;

3) A review of the use of restrictions and procedures over the past thirty (30) days noting frequency, duration, location, time frames and individuals and staff members involved;

4) An observation of the resident on at least two (2) occasions in those areas and at those times suggestions by the above analysis to be the most likely for the targeted behaviors to occur;

5) A discussion with staff members working with the residents behavior;

6) An analysis of the data and observations to include;

A. A summary of data and observations,

B. An analysis of and hypothesis of the events causing a particular behavior and what re-enforcers are maintaining the behavior;

C. Make recommendations regarding the environment and type of behavior plan.

When the team embarks on writing the behavior management plan the following four (4) points must always be considered:

1) When a behavioral barrier or barriers have been defined;

2) When goals and objectives are identified;

3) When the use of a restrictive procedure being implemented exceeds the limit approved by the treatment team;

4) When the use of an emergency procedure exceeds the limit stipulated and approved by the treatment team and professional staff.

When writing a behavior management plan attention must always first be given to the medical treatment being provided to address purely medical etiologies, physical or occupational therapies, or environmental manipulations which may preclude the need for a behavioral management plan. And all behavioral plans should be written within one (1) week after the interdisciplinary team has identified existing barriers and programmatic needs. Any member of the treatment team may write a behavior management plan and develop a method of recording and tracking data. When writing a behavioral management plan the team members should make every effort to insure that all behavior techniques utilized during the procedure emphasize the following:

1) Positive approaches;

2) Employ the least restrictive measures available;

3) Maintain the least intrusive approaches possible; and

4) Insure that all behavior management plans are temporary in nature.

When assessing data obtained during comprehensive evaluation the team members should remember to:

1) Consider what the resident can do;

2) What the resident will do; and

3) What the resident may do.

When team members utilize data obtained during assessment they should:

1) Keep the plan, goals and objectives positive, specific, simple and doable;

2) Select a strategy;

3) Make the process a team effort;

4) Plan, do, and review;

5) Evaluate and re-evaluate;

6) Make adjustments if and when necessary.

When developing a behavior plan to change behavior remind team members that the plan should be implemented with:

a) Patience;

b) Careful observation;

c) Time;

d) Hard work; and

e) Consistency.

When implementing any behavioral management plan it must receive sign – off signatures of the following:

1) Administrator of Facility;

2) Medical Director;

3) Director of Nursing;

4) Team Members;

5) Responsible Family Member or Legal Guardian;

6) Resident Advocate/Ombudsman.

When participating in the evaluation process team members should address the following questions:

1) Does plan solicit and value family input?

2) Are existing support systems being involved?

3) Is programming technically sound?

4) Is plan being administered in a humane fashion? And

5) Is all programming being done in accordance with all legal and ethical standards of federal, state and society.

The team responsible for developing the plan must adhere to the principle that behavior modification is a teaching procedure. It does not attempt to explain dementia, Alzheimer's Disease, inappropriate or disruptive behavior associated with the condition. The aim of behavior modification is a positive one which focuses on changing and producing improvement in the residents inappropriate behavior rather than assuming a passive role of merely observing and giving explanations. It should place emphasis on and focus on the following principles: 1) that all behavior is caused, 2) that behavior is not a fixed characteristic of an individual, and 3) that behavior can be changed if the causes are defined and changed in order to accomplish therapeutic gains. The success of behavior modification rests upon careful attention and arrangement of the consequences of behavior since it occurs mainly because of the effects which it produces. Therefore, change in behavior is most easily produced by careful arrangement of the consequences of behavior. Thus, it is this rather simple fact that behavior modification is established.

The treatment team is never finished with eliminating an undesirable behavior until a socially appropriate response is achieved. So, after the team has eliminated an undesirable behavior they should move on to the next step of producing a socially appropriate response. It is a matter of replacing a socially inappropriate response with a socially appropriate one.

In conclusion, a hierarchy of treatment for the elderly suffering from Alzheimer's Dementia for managing their disruptive and aggressive behavior should be implemented using the most benign and comfortable procedures first. The first hierarchy should include treatment procedures which include training programs which involve reinforcement, meaningful and interesting activities which are therapeutic throughout the residents waking hours.

The second hierarchy of treatment should be introduced to augment the first. This should consist of a loss of something important and meaningful to the resident such as privileges. Many times behavior problems can be eliminated during such training activities by preventing the negative behavior from occurring in the first place. If progress is slow or fails to respond to the first and second hierarchies of treatment the third hierarchy should be introduced which emphasizes the use of a quite area, removal from the group, time out, required relaxation and positive practice. All three of these hierarchies emphasize: 1) positive approaches, 2) least restrictive measures available, 3) the least intrusive approaches, and 4) are temporary in nature.

The following enclosures are examples of behavior management plans which have been written and implemented in long term care facilities to assist in or augment existing treatment procedures for managing disruptive and aggressive behavior in their facilities. All are written utilizing the preceding hierarchies of treatment.

BEHAVIOR MANAGEMENT PLAN

EXAMPLE

Resident _____ Age _____ Record No. _____

Responsible Staff Member_____

Living Area

Date of BMP_____

Date Implemented_____

The persons listed below attended the special team meeting held on

_____

for _____ for the purpose of Developing

a BEHAVIOR MANAGEMENT PLAN.

I.   BASIS FOR BEHAVIORAL INTERVENTION:

       A.   Resident receiving psychotropic medication.

       B.   Resident exhibiting inappropriate behavior.

II. PROCEDURE: Resident will be rewarded for appropriate and/or

desired behavior by using verbal, gestural, and physical prompts. The resident will never be rewarded by any method when exhibiting inappropriate or undesired behavior. Liquids and edibles may be used if prior approval is obtained from medical and dietary staff. Always give resident an explanation of why a reward is being given. Residents progress or lack of it, changes, modification, deletion, or termination of program will be documented in the residents record and reflected in progress notes.

Signature   Title

_____   _____

_____   _____

_____   _____

_____   _____

_____   _____

_____   _____

_____   _____

III. SUBJECT: Rummaging.

IV. GOAL: To reduce occurrences of rummaging.

V. OBJECTIVE: Mr. Rummage will reduce his incidences of rummaging to four (4) or less per month by_____.

VI. DEFINITION OF BEHAVIOR (RUMMAGING).

A compulsive and/or ritualistic pattern of both day and night roams during which time the resident gets out of bed before going to sleep or wakes up from sleep and wanders about the building engaging in behavior which often awakens, disturbs, or agitates others by going through the personal belongings of others taking or attempting to take things and objects for no apparent reason or purpose.

VII. METHOD: When resident is seen rummaging, the staff member will:

Steps:

1. Approach the resident in a calm and non-threatening manner. The staff member will make and hold eye contact remaining kind, gentle and giving verbal reinforcement and reassurance as needed to keep from further frightening the resident.

2. The staff member will with minimal hands-on approach, gently take the resident by the arm and redirect and/or guide him or her back to room, living or assigned area refraining from scolding or starting to participate in an argument.

3. If the resident refuses to cooperate, the staff member will call for assistance from another staff member and when positioned on each side of the resident, gently grasp each arm and walk and/or guide back to room, living or assigned area giving verbal reinforcement reassuring the resident while doing so.

4. The preceding sequences will be repeated as often as necessary. If resident continues to rummage, exhibit disruptive and non-compliant behavior, contact professional in charge for consultation.

5. The staff will, in consultation with medical or professional in charge, label all personal belongings with resident's name, and provide resident with a box containing personal belongings to rummage through to prevent and further control resident's rummaging.

6. If rummaging continues repeat steps 1 through 5 for four (4) times and then consult with medical and professional staff for further instructions.

III. SUBJECT: mood disorder, depression.

IV. GOAL: to reduce incidents of depression.

V. OBJECTIVE: Ms. Doe will reduce her episodes of depression by decreasing the behavioral causes, (non-compliance), which contribute to her incidents of depression (failing to follow directions, procedures, and requests) to two (2) or less occurrences per month by _____

VI. DEFINITION OF BEHAVIORAL CAUSES: Withdrawal from activities and social events (isolation by preferring to stay in room and refusing to participate in meals in the dining room). A deterioration of or loss of interests and a lack of cooperation and performance among peers and staff.

VII. METHOD:

Day 1 – A. Staff member will politely knock and enter residents room and patiently explain in detail the team concept, philosophy and expectations of its residents and how she as a resident is to be an active participant in all activities provided by the treatment team and facility. Staff member will explain to her that all programs and activities are scheduled for the sole purpose of enriching and improving her lifestyle. And more importantly such activities are planned to assist her in achieving and maintaining good physical, mental and emotional health which in the final analysis will assure her a better quality of life. If resident makes no effort to respond, staff will say your behavior is not acceptable and leave room without any kind of verbal, gestural, or physical reward.

Day 2 – B. When it is time to wake up, a staff member will politely knock on Ms. Doe's door and enter her room and in a kind but firm voice, say, "Ms. Doe, it is time to get up and get dressed for breakfast". If she is non-compliant the staff member will repeat Step A and add, "Your behavior is not acceptable" and leave room without giving reward.

Day 3 – C. If Ms. Doe continues to refuse to cooperate the staff member will, in a kind but firm manner, show a force of authority. Staff member will accomplish this by exhibiting a stiff and determined body posture, a kind but firm voice when speaking, by making and holding eye contact, maintaining rigid facial expressions and attitude to convey to Ms. Doe his/her position of strength, determination and authority as opposed to one of weakness. The staff member will repeat steps A & B, and leave room immediately without giving reward..

Day 4 – D. If Ms. Doe continues to be non-compliant, the staff member will repeat steps A, B and C, and will then with minimum physical hands-on approach assist Ms. Doe with toileting, grooming, and dressing and then gently take her by the arm and direct/or guide her out of her room and on to the dining area. The staff member will in a kind but firm manner maintain a posture of structure and determination rewarding Ms. Doe verbally if she begins to cooperate. Repeat steps A, B, & C, if necessary.

Day 5 – E. If Ms. Doe continues to be defiant the staff member will call for assistance and the two staff members will, after repeating steps A, B, C, and D, approach Ms. Doe in a calm and non-threatening manner making and holding eye contact while at the same time remaining kind and gentle giving her verbal reinforcement and reassurance as needed to keep from frightening her. The staff members will position themselves on each side of Ms. Doe and using their bodies and minimum hands-on control, gently grasp her arms and slowly begin to escort/guide her from her room to the dining room area giving her verbal reinforcements as they do so.

Day 6 – F. When arriving at designated dining area, the staff will congratulate Ms. Doe on her accomplishment continuing to use verbal commands and minimal hands-on control using their bodies to show her directions, giving verbal reinforcement, and encouragement to re-assure her. When dining is completed, the staff will escort Ms. Doe back to her room using minimum hands-on control giving her verbal, gestural and physical reinforcement while doing so. If she complains about staff interfering simply state in a kind but firm manner, "Ms. Doe, when you can get up, get dressed and do these activities on your own, we will cease assisting you—and that will be great."

G. If resident can independently perform objective (getting up, getting dressed, and going to and from dining room) the staff will gradually withdraw their direct intervention but will continue to reward resident for appropriate/desired behavior by giving verbal, gestural and physical prompts/rewards.

H. The staff will repeat the above sequences A through F, as often as necessary in consultation with appropriate medical and professional personnel to achieve and maintain compliance in appropriate social interaction and cooperation.

III. SUBJECT: Sleep Problems – Staying awake at night.

IV. GOAL: To reduce staying awake.

V. OBJECTIVE: Ms. Slumber will reduce occurrences of staying awake at night to ten (10) incidents or less per month by _____.

VI. DEFINITION OF BEHAVIOR (STAYING AWAKE AT NIGHT): Defined as exhibiting a problem, habit or develops a routine of staying awake at night.

VII. METHOD: When resident has a problem, habit or develops a routine of staying awake at night, the staff will:

STEPS:

1. Provide resident with regular periods of exercise and reduce/delete daytime napping or sleeping.

2. Delete all foods or drinks containing caffeine from the residents late afternoon and evening menus.

3. Develop a routine for the use of the bathroom with the resident, use a night light, or extra lighting at night in room; make a safe pathway to the bathroom or use a bedside commode.

4. Permit the resident to have a bedtime snack for hunger.

5. Create a bedtime routine that is soothing and relaxing to the resident, i.e. soft listening music, non-aggressive/exciting T.V. programs, or a glass of warm milk to help resident wind down.

6. Avoid letting resident go to bed too early.

7. Allow resident to sleep in recliner in room or near nursing station if desired to promote a feeling of security. OR if resident must be up at night, provide supervision.

8. If resident continues to have occurrences after these steps are implemented, the staff will: Reorient the resident to time, place and person emphasizing that night is a time for sleep and doing so by comforting and reassuring the resident emphasizing safety and security using a quite soothing tone of voice giving verbal reinforcement and touch.

9. If the resident insists on getting out of bed or making loud noises, the staff member will guide the resident out of the room to an area where other residents will not be disturbed into a well lighted area.

10. The staff member will guide the resident close to a nursing station providing interaction or activities that will help occupy resident's time such as providing boxes of interesting objects of textiles encourag-

ing the resident to perform repetitive tasks like folding clothes or linen and providing music by earphones, using T.V. or giving a snack.

11. The above sequence may be repeated as often as necessary. If the resident does not respond by developing appropriate sleep habits seek assistance from professional in charge and schedule a team meeting.

II. SUBJECT: Fighting

IV. GOAL: Reduce Episodes of Fighting.

V. OBJECTIVE: Ms. Flippant will reduce incidents of fighting to one (1) or less occurrences per month by _____.

VI. DEFINITION OF FIGHTING: Self-initiated behavior making bodily contact with another person with his or her fist, open hand, arms, or foot attacking him or her by striking, scratching, choking, pinching, biting, cutting, pulling hair, or by throwing objects at him or her with no provocation from the other person.

VII. METHOD: When resident begins fighting, the staff member will:

STEPS:

1. Assume a posture of authority characterized by a determined approach, a loud, stern, but kind voice when speaking, making and holding eye contact, firm and rigid facial expressions, kind but firm mannerisms to show a position of strength, determination and control as opposed to one of weakness and say "stop". "This behavior is not appropriate and will not be tolerated".

2. Give a loud, strong and firm verbal command to stop fighting – making and holding eye contact and using body and hands-on control to stop fighting.

3. Separate and redirect away from individual or group to a quite area, giving resident personal space, remaining a safe distance from resident, giving the opportunity to calm down, using verbal interaction and touch to further calm, informing resident what is and is not acceptable behavior.

4. If not able to calm resident and for protection, get out of range of resident or leave area, providing the resident is safe, giving the resident an opportunity to calm down.

5. If resident continues to be combative, solicit help from another staff member for assistance using firm, verbal reinforcement, touch, and give the resident comfort objects such as a doll or stuffed animal to calm and reassure always giving resident the sense that you are in control.

6. If procedure fails, repeat steps 1, 2, 3, 4 and 5, for four (4) consecutive times and if resident remains combative, call professional in charge for consultation. Schedule a team meeting.

III.   SUBJECT: Aggression.

IV.   GOAL: To reduce aggression.

V. OBJECTIVE: Mr. Slap will reduce his incidents of aggressive behavior to ten (10) or less occurrences per month by _____.

VI. DEFINITION OF BEHAVIOR (AGGRESSIVE) exhibits verbal, physical aggression, cursing, spitting, screaming, hitting, slapping, biting, or violating the privacy of others.

VII. METHOD: Whenever resident exhibits behavior defined as aggression, the staff member will:

STEPS:

1. Assume position of authority and say, "Stop", in a firm, loud voice, after making eye contact to gain attention, tell the resident that this behavior is not appropriate and will not be tolerated and ask resident to please make an effort to explain why; such behavior is being exhibited.

2. If necessary, physically interrupt the behavior and prompt resident to instead exhibit behavior appropriate to the current program or activity.

3. If resident continues to exhibit aggressive behavior, remove resident to quite area away from the group until calm for five (5) minutes. If necessary, use minimal amount of hands-on contact necessary to prevent resident from leaving assigned or quite area.

4. After resident has completed five (5) minutes of calmness, prompt resident to return to group and resume normal activity.

5. If resident again begins to exhibit aggressive and inappropriate behavior, repeat steps 1, 2, 3 & 4.

6. If resident remains aggressive after steps 1, 2, 3 & 4 have been repeated four (4) times, a professional will be consulted to determine further action and schedule team meeting.

III. SUBJECT: Assault.

IV. GOAL: To reduce assault.

V. OBJECTIVE: Mr. Fling will reduce his assault to five (5) or less occurrences per month by _____.

VI. DEFINITION OF ASSAULT: Any type of hitting, biting, pinching, slapping, scratching, throwing objects at, or attempting to exhibit such behavior.

VII. METHOD: When Mr. Fling begins to exhibit behavior defined as assault, the staff will:

STEPS:

1. Assume a posture of authority by exhibiting an aloof and determined image characterized by speaking in a loud but firm manner, maintaining a matter-of-fact attitude, making and holding eye contact with firm and rigid facial expressions, maintaining kind but firm mannerisms showing a force of authority and control conveying his or her position of strength, determination, and authority as opposed to one of weakness and say, "stop, your behavior is inappropriate".

2. The staff member will say "stop" in a loud but firm voice and with gestural and physical prompts direct Mr. Fling to become involved in an activity appropriate to the current schedule.

3. If behavior does not subside, staff will call for assistance from another staff member and position on each side of Mr. Fling, taking him by each arm, and escort/guide/walk him to his room or to quite area away from group and remain with him. If he remains calm and non-assaultive for five (5) minutes reward him with verbal, gestural and physical prompts and return him to group or assigned area.

4. If Mr. Fling remains assaultive after steps 1 through 3 have been repeated four (4) times, call and consult medical and professional staff for further instructions. Schedule team meeting.

III. SUBJECT: Self-Abuse.

IV. GOAL: To reduce self-abuse.

V. OBJECTIVE: Ms. Trooper will reduce her incidents of self-abuse to two (2) or less occurrences per month by _____.

VI. DEFINITION OF SELF-ABUSE: Intentional use of force to harm and/or inflict damage or injury to one's self (slapping, hitting, biting, banging one's face, or body harshly).

VII. METHOD: When resident is self-abusing, the staff member will:

STEPS:

1. When Ms. Trooper begins to exhibit behavior defined as self-abuse, the staff will assume a posture of authority by taking a stance of being aloof and determined image, speaking in a firm, loud voice, maintaining a matter-of-fact attitude, making and holding eye contact, maintain rigid and firm facial expressions, kind and firm manner-isms, showing a force of authority and control conveying a position of strength, determination, and authority as opposed to one of weakness. Staff member will give resident a strong verbal command to "Stop

abusive behavior". "Your behavior is not appropriate and will not be tolerated".

2. If resident continues, walk and redirect away from area giving verbal, gestural and physical gestures and using the minimum hands-on control to touch, rub, pat, and stroke to calm and to halt abusive behavior for five (5) minutes.

3. If the behavior continues, repeat the above procedure for four (4) times.

4. After the procedure is repeated for four (4) times and the resident remains self-abusive, the professional in charge should be contacted for consultation. A team meeting will be scheduled.

III. SUBJECT: Non-compliance.

IV. GOAL: To reduce behavior (non-compliance).

V. OBJECTIVE: Mr. Boss will reduce his non-compliance to ten (10) or less occurrences per month by _____.

VI. DEFINITION OF BEHAVIOR (NON-COMPLIANCE): Failing to follow directions or procedures.

VII. METHOD: When staff observes a resident exhibiting non-compliant behavior:

STEPS:

1. When resident exhibits non-compliant behavior, the staff member will assume a posture of strength and determination, and, in a loud but firm voice, say "stop, your behavior is not acceptable".

2. If the resident continues to be non-compliant gently place your hand on the resident's arm and redirect to an area away from where non-compliant behavior is being exhibited for five (5) minutes.

3. After resident completes five (5) minutes of calm behavior, resident will be allowed to return to previous area and resume normal activities.

4. If resident again becomes non-compliant repeat steps 1, 2, & 3.

5. If resident remains non-compliant after steps 1, 2, 3, & 4 have been repeated four (4) times, then contact and consult with professional in charge and schedule team meeting.

III. SUBJECT: Verbal abuse.

IV. GOAL: To reduce verbal abuse.

V. OBJECTIVE: Ms. Mouthy will reduce her incidents of verbal abuse to ten (10) or less occurrences per month by _____.

VI. DEFINITION OF BEHAVIOR (VERBAL ABUSE): Cursing, swearing, spitting, yelling or screaming.

VII. METHOD: When Ms. Mouthy begins to exhibit behavior defined as verbal abuse, the staff will:

STEPS:

1. Assume a posture of authority, say "Stop", in a firm loud voice and the prompt the resident instead to become involved in an activity appropriate to the current schedule. If resident continues to exhibit verbal abuse, the staff member will:

2. Take resident to an area away from the group, i. e. to a "quite area" and prompt the resident to remain there until calm for two (2) minutes.

3. If resident is not calm within thirty (30) minutes, or is so disruptive that the safety of resident and others cannot be ensured using separation from the group, repeat steps 1, 2, & 3.

4. If resident remains verbal abusive after steps 1, 2, & 3 have been repeated four (4) times, then call and consult professional in charge. Schedule team meeting.

III. SUBJECT: Wandering.

IV. GOAL: To reduce wandering.

V. OBJECTIVE: Mr. Yonder will reduce his incidents of wandering to five (5) or less occurrences per month or less by _____.

VI. DEFINITION: Consistently leaving group, room or assigned area without permission exhibiting "hyperactivity" like or "escape" type behavior such as persistently walking aimlessly about facility, fleeting from task to task or from activity to activity without a sense of direction. Behavior (wandering) may not be functional and may appear to be movements for the sake of movement.

VII. METHOD: When staff observes a resident leaving assigned area and beginning to wander, the staff shall:

STEPS:

1. Approach resident from the side or in front.

2. Gently using verbal commands and minimal hands-on control, redirect the resident back to assigned area using your body to show direction.

3. Distract resident from their wandering by talking about a favorite topic, or focusing their attention on something else while guiding back to assigned area—give verbal reinforcement, encouragement and touch to reassure.

4. If resident does not respond to the staff members effort to redirect back into assigned area, let the resident finish or complete that which is being attempted, remaining with the resident to ensure safety. Wait until resident is open to other suggestions or alternatives and guide back into facility or assigned area reminding resident which is and is not acceptable.

5. If resident continues to be resistant, detain and call for the assistance of another staff member. Each staff member will position themselves on each side of the resident and using their bodies and minimum hands-on control, gently grasp the residents arms to escort and guide the resident back into building or assigned area giving verbal reinforcement.

6. If all attempts fail to return resident to assigned area, repeat procedure up to four (4) times and then call professional in charge for consultation. Schedule team meeting.

III. SUBJECT: Yelling

IV. GOAL: To decrease episodes of yelling.

V. OBJECTIVE: Ms. Nillie will reduce her incidences of yelling to four (4) or less occurrences for month by _____.

VI. DEFINITION OF YELLING: An emission of repetitive, inappropriate, irrelevant, stereotyped, and disruptive verbalizations or sounds, not due to a lack of speech, for reasons other than a reaction to obvious painful stimuli.

VII. METHOD:

STEPS:

1. Whenever Ms. Nillie has an episode of yelling the staff member will assume a posture of authority. This will be done by displaying an aloof and determined image, speaking in a loud, but firm matter of fact voice, making and holding eye contact, maintaining firm and rigid facial expressions along with kind but firm mannerisms to show a force of authority covering his or her position of strength, determination and authority as opposed to one of weakness.

2. Staff member will repeat step 1 + say, "Ms. Nillie", in a loud but firm voice "stop your yelling" in a matter of fact manner giving no positive reinforcement.

3. If Ms. Nillie continues to yell the staff member will repeat steps 1 and 2, intervene and remove any objects Ms. Nillie is aggressive towards from reach and redirect her away from group to her room or to a quite area until she is calm for five (5) minutes. This will be done in a matter of fact manner with no positive reinforcement.

4. If Ms. Nillie continues to yell the staff member will repeat 1, 2, & 3, and intervene requesting assistance from another staff member to stop the behavior by using hands-on control to escort Ms. Nillie to an area away from group where she can be alone but observed. The staff should avoid all eye contact, all interaction including communication during this procedure. The staff will give no positive reinforcements.

5. If Ms. Nillie continues to yell the staff will repeat steps 1, 2, 3, & 4, and will observe from a distance but closely monitoring. Check every fifteen (15) minutes to monitor for health and safety reasons in consultation with medical and professional staff. Avoid giving any type of verbal, gestural or physical rewards, ignore behavior, maintain matter of fact attitude.

6. If Ms. Nillie continues to yell repeat steps 1 through 5 and begin frequency count of number of yells per minute. Reward with verbal, gestural, and physical prompts for decrease in frequency of yelling.

7. If Ms. Nillie decreases her frequency of yelling reward with immediate attention giving verbal, gestural, and physical prompts, and move her back to group or assigned area. Continue to give positive rewards with individual attention.

8. Repeat steps 1 through 7 as often as necessary to achieve objective. Yelling is often a means of demanding and getting attention. As these needs are met yelling often subsides. If above procedure fails call medical and professional staff for further attention and schedule team meeting for further action.

III. SUBJECT: Hoarding..

IV. GOAL: To reduce incidences of hoarding.

V. OBJECTIVE: Ms. Wingit will reduce her occurrences of hoarding to five (5) or less incidents per month by _____.

VI. DEFINITION: A compulsive and ritualistic pattern of both day and night roams during which time the resident wanders about the building, unit or rooms engaging in unacceptable behavior of collecting, keeping and hiding a large number of things or objects which do not belong to him or her and hiding/hoarding them for no apparent reason or purpose.

VII. METHOD: When resident is hoarding, the staff member will:

STEPS:

1. Approach the resident in a calm and non-threatening manner. The staff member will make and hold eye contact remaining kind, gentle and giving verbal reinforcement and reassurance as needed to keep from further frightening the resident.

2. The staff member will with minimal hands-on approach, gently take the resident by the arm and redirect and/or guide the resident back

233

to room, living or assigned area refraining from scolding or starting to participate in an argument.

3. If the resident refuses to cooperate the staff member will call for assistance from another staff member and when positioned on each side of the resident, gently grasp each arm and walk and/or guide back to room, living or assigned area giving verbal reinforcement reassuring the resident while doing so.

4. The preceding sequences will be repeated as often as necessary. If resident continues to hoard, exhibit disruptive and on-compliant behavior, contact professional in charge for consultation.

5. The staff will, in consultation with professional in charge, identify favorite hiding places, label all personal belongings with resident's name, and provide resident with a box containing personal belongings to rummage through to prevent and further control resident's hoarding.

6. If resident continues to hoard, repeat steps 1 through 3 and call team meeting to further deal with behavior of hoarding.

CHAPTER THIRTEEN

FORMS FOR RECORDING DATA

Whatever form is selected for use to report data, it should reflect the trainers direct observation of the residents behavior. The trainer should try to observe the residents performance and/or behavior in a natural setting. Data should be collected constantly, randomly, or at scheduled intervals depending on the situation. For example, if the only one taking data on several residents in a group, the observations must be either a random or at scheduled times unless the trainer has other staff members assisting in taking data. However, when the trainer is taking data alone in a one-to-one situation the trainer can observe the resident constantly. Also an experienced and skilled trainer is able to train and keep records at the same time.

There are two kinds of evaluation which must be done and on which data must be kept when training a resident(s): 1) process evaluation and 2) produce evaluation. Process evaluation is when data is recorded to see if strategies are working. Produce evaluation is done to see whether or not objectives are being met. Recording and tracking data provides the trainer with a permanent record of training methods and accomplishments. Such records are necessary for future training programs; they are also necessary to the facility for funding and conformity with Federal and State regulations.

The trainer may choose to record data in one of the following ways: charts, graphs, either bar or line, attendance records, narrative notes on daily activities, or by established observation. Also, it might be appropriate to use a combination of these forms. Then, too, there are times when the trainer will want to design forms on which to record data and adapt them to his or her own needs. Whatever the case, all forms should be kept simple. The following are some examples of forms used to record data during the training process.

VERBAL CONSENT
EXAMPLE

Name_____

Number_____

AUTHORIZATION TO USE RESTRICTIVE OR INTRUSIVE
PROCEDURES IN CONJUNCTION WITH A BEHAVIOR MANAGEMENT PLAN

I, the responsible party for _____, have read the proposed Behavior Management Plan which was developed and approved by an interdisciplinary team and dated _____, and which is intended to teach _____more socially acceptable behavior.

I agree that this plan is in the best interest of _____ and should be implemented accordingly. I hereby authorize _____ (name of nursing center) professional staff to employ the use of

_____-

_____(Specify Restrictive or Intrusive Procedures) as written in the Behavior Management Plan under prescribed conditions.

I am aware that I can withdraw this consent at any time, except to the extent that action has been taken in reliance thereon.

_____	_____
Signature of Resident	Person Giving Verbal Consent
_____	_____
Date	Relationship to Above-Named Individual
	_____
	Date
_____	
Witness	
_____	
Date	

James W. Ramage Ph.D.

VERBAL CONSENT
EXAMPLE

Name_____

Number_____

AUTHORIZATION TO USE RESTRICTIVE OR INTRUSIVE
PROCEDURES IN CONJUNCTION WITH A BEHAVIOR MANAGEMENT PLAN

    I, the responsible party for _____, have read
the proposed Behavior Management Plan which was developed and approved by an
interdisciplinary team and dated _____, and which is intended to teach
_____more socially acceptable behavior.

    I agree that this plan is in the best interest of _____
and should be implemented accordingly. I hereby authorize _____
(name of nursing center) professional staff to employ the use of

_____-

_____(Specify Restrictive or
Intrusive Procedures) as written in the Behavior Management Plan under prescribed
conditions.

    I am aware that I can withdraw this consent at any time, except to the extent that
action has been taken in reliance thereon.

_____   _____
Signature of Resident   Person Giving Verbal Consent

_____   _____
Date   Relationship to Above-Named Individual

    _____
    Date

_____
Witness

_____
Date

CONSENT FOR THE USE OF NEUROLEPTIC MEDICATIONS
EXAMPLE

RESIDENT NAME_____

RECORD NUMBER_____

Neuroleptic medication is a medication which is prescribed for the purpose of treating a psychiatric disorder or modifying behavior.

All neuroleptics are prescribed using accepted dosage guidelines.

Although this doesn't happen often, data from research shows that some individuals taking neuroleptics have undesirable side effects such as muscle spasms or tremors (which clear up when the medication is stopped or the dosage reduced). Even less frequently, involuntary movements of the face, mouth, tongue, limbs, and trunk may occur and do not clear as quickly or become permanent. This is called tardive dyskinesia.

We want to inform you that there is a possibility of such side effects when one takes neuroleptic medication, but the team feels that in this case the benefits of the medication far outweigh the risks.

The team feels that _____would benefit from neuroleptic medication due to the following diagnosis or behaviors: _____.

PHYSICIAN:_____DATE:_____
                    Signature

I have read the above information and approve the use of neuroleptic medications within accepted dosage ranges as described above and as utilized as a part of _____ Behavior Modification Plan.

_____   _____

Signature of Resident, Legal Guardian,   Date
or Next-of-kin

_____

Relationship to Resident

_____   _____

Witness if Resident Signed   Date

This consent may be REVOKED IN WRITING at any time except to the extent that action has been taken thereon. If not specifically revoked, this consent will be in effect from _____(date) to _____(date).

James W. Ramage Ph.D.

INDIVIDUAL THERAPEUTIC ACTIVITY PLAN
EXAMPLE Page 1

Resident_____ Age_____ Record No. _____

Date of ITAP _____ Date Completed _____ Date Implemented_____

    The persons listed below attended team meeting held on _____ for
:_____ for the purpose of developing an individual
therapeutic activity plan and doing so with maximum involvement of attending team
members, the resident and family members alike. This activity plan was developed
individualized, tailored to and written to define, target and address a specific need or
needs of _____ following comprehensive assessments to include
behavioral, medical, recreational, social and functional analysis.

    The method of implementing plan will consist of resident(s) being rewarded by
trainer when exhibiting desired and or appropriate behavior by using verbal, gestural, and
physical prompts. Activities will also serve as reinforcers such as sitting in a special
chair, going for a ride or walk, watching a movie, etc. In addition, liquids and edibles
are also used as reinforcers when approved by medical and dietary staff. The resident(s)
will always be given an explanation of why a reward is being given. All progress or lack
of it will be documented and reflected in progress notes.

    The plan will be implemented by trained and supervised staff in a technically sound,
humane and non-intrusive manner as possible in accordance with all legal and ethical
standards of society.

Signature   Title

_____   _____

_____   _____

_____   _____

_____   _____

_____   _____

_____   _____

_____   _____

_____   _____

_____   _____

_____   _____

INDIVIDUAL THERAPEUTIC ACTIVITY PLAN (ITAP)

Name _____ Date _____ Room No. _____

Resident Participated in Developing Activity Plan: Yes _____ No _____ Comments_____

Family Participated in Developing Plan: Yes __ No __ Comments_____

Strengths   Needs

_____   _____
_____   _____
_____   _____
_____   _____

Prioritized I Goals   Prioritized II Goals

_____   _____
_____   _____
_____   _____

Schedule: Days _____ Times _____ Trainer(s) _____
                        (Circle Assigned Group)

Group A	Group B	Group C
(a) Mild Skill Loss	(a) Moderate Skill Loss	(a) Severe Skill Loss
(b) In Room Activity	(b) In Room Activity	(b) In Room Activity
(c) In Assigned Area	(c) In Assigned Area	(c) In Assigned Area
(d) In Large Group	(d) In Large/Small Group	(d) In Small Group
(e) Other _____	(e) Other _____	(e) Other _____

Interest, Requirement or Need: (Check Appropriately): Social _____ Religious _____
Indoor _____ Outdoor _____ Creative _____ Music _____ Educational _____ Relaxation _____
Cognitive _____ Esteem Building _____ Exercise _____ Outings _____ Self Help Skills _____
ADL's _____ Psychological _____ Other (Explain) _____

Special Directions: _____
_____

Strategy: (who, when, how) _____
_____

Therapeutic Purpose of Activity: _____

Barrier _____   Solution _____
Barrier _____   Solution _____

Process Evaluation Done: _____
Post Evaluation Done: Date _____ Results _____

Approved By: _____   Completed By: _____
              Consultant   Title

James W. Ramage Ph.D.

INDIVIDUAL THERAPEUTIC ACTIVITY PLAN
GOALS AND OBJECTIVES
EXAMPLE

Resident _____ Program _____

Goal 1 _____

Objective 1.1 _____

_____

Date Started _____ Date Ended _____

Reason Obj. Ended _____

Rationale For Change _____

Signature of Trainer _____

Objective 1.2 _____

_____

Date Started _____ Date Ended _____

Reason Obj. Ended _____

Rationale For Change _____

Signature of Trainer _____

Objective 1.3 _____

_____

Date Started _____ Date Ended _____

Reason Obj. Ended _____

Rationale For Change _____

Signature of Trainer _____

Objective 1.4 _____

_____

Date Started _____ Date Ended _____

Reason Obj. Ended _____

Rationale For Change _____

Signature of Trainer _____

Objective: 1.5 _____

_____

Date Started _____ Date Ended _____

Reason Obj. Ended _____

Rationale For Change _____

Signature of Trainer _____

INDIVIDUAL THERAPEUTIC ACTIVITY PLAN
GOALS AND OBJECTIVES
EXAMPLE

Resident _____ Program _____
Goal 2 _____

Objective 2.1 _____
_____

Date Started _____ Date Ended _____
Reason Obj. Ended _____
Rationale For Change _____
Signature of Trainer _____

Objective 2.2 _____
_____

Date Started _____ Date Ended _____
Reason Obj. Ended _____
Rationale For Change _____
Signature of Trainer _____

Objective 2.3 _____
_____

Date Started _____ Date Ended _____
Reason Obj. Ended _____
Rationale For Change _____
Signature of Trainer _____

Objective 2.4 _____
_____

Date Started _____ Date Ended _____
Reason Obj. Ended _____
Rationale For Change _____
Signature of Trainer _____

Objective 2.5 _____
_____

Date Started _____ Date Ended _____
Reason Obj. Ended _____
Rationale For Change _____
Signature of Trainer _____

James W. Ramage Ph.D.

ASSESSMENT OF PROGRESS
EXAMPLE

Resident:_____ Date of ITAP _____
PROGRESS MADE SINCE LAST INDIVIDUAL THERAPEUTIC ACTIVITY
PLAN (ITAP) MEETING

Date	Goal/Obj.#	Program Name	Begun	Ended	Progress

QUALITATIVE
DATA SHEET   **Behavior Modification Assessment Instrument**

INSTRUCTIONS: Rate the task using the score key below. In addition,
 If a physical prompt is needed, record a P.
 If a gestural prompt is needed, record a G.
 If a verbal prompt is needed, record a V.

SCORE KEY: (A) no response   (D) good approximation
               (B) incorrect response   (E) excellent approximation
               (C) poor approximation   (F) can generalize to natural environment

RESIDENTS NAME:_____   TRAINERS NAME_____

DATE	TASK /STEPS							SCORE									

REMARKS:

BASELINE DATA SHEET

RESIDENT _____RECORD NUMBER _____

DATE _____ LIVING AREA _____

TARGET BEHAVIORS; 1) _____

_____

_____

_____

2) _____

_____

_____

Time	1STBehavior	2nd Behavior	Ini	Time	1ST Behavior	2ND Behavior	Ini
6:00				2:00			
6:30				2:30			
7:00				3:00			
7:30				3:30			
8:00				4:00			
8:30				4:30			
9:00				5:00			
9:30				5:30			
10:00				6:00			
10:30				6:30			
11:00				7:00			
11:30				7:30			
12:00				8:00			
12:30				8:30			
1:00				9:00			
1:30				9:30			

DAILY TRAINING LOG

TRAINER _____ DATE _____

RESIDENT'S NAME _____

TASK	TIME BEGAN	TIME ENDED	TOTAL TIME	TOTAL NUMBER OF TRIALS

COMMENTS _____
_____
_____
_____

James W. Ramage Ph.D.

WEEKLY TRAINING SUMMARY

TRAINER _____ DATE _____

RESIDENT'S NAME _____

TASK	NUMBER OF TIMES TRAINED	RANGE OF TRAINING INTERVAL	AVERAGE TRAINING INTERVAL	AVERAGE NUMBER TRIALS

COMMENTS_____
_____
_____
_____

248

MONTHLY PROGRESS NOTES

LAST NAME   FIRST NAME   ROOM NO.   ATTENDING PHYSICIAN

DATE	TIME	NOTES SHOULD BE SIGNED

REFERENCES

Abeles, N. (ed.) (1997). What Practitioners Should Know about Working with Older Adults. Washington, D.C.: American Psychological Association.

Allain, H., Schuck S., Ferrer, D.B., Bourin, M., Vercelletto M., Reymann, J.M., Polard E., Anxiolytics in the Treatment of Behavioral and Psychological Symptoms of Dementia International Psychogeriatrics, Vol. 12, Suppl. 1.

Alzheimer Caregiver's Handbook (2003). Alzheimer's Foundation of the South Mississippi Division. Gulfport, Ms.

American Psychiatric Association. (1994). Diagnostic and Statistical Manual of Mental Disorders, 4th ed. Washington, D.C.: American Psychiatric Association.

American Psychiatric Association, (1997). Practice Guideline for the Treatment of Patients with Alzheimer's Disease and Other Dementias of Late Life. Washington, D.C.: American Psychiatric Association.

American Psychological Association. (1990). Guidelines for Providers of Psychological Services to Ethnic, Linguistic, and Culturally Diverse Populations. Washington, D.C.: American Psychological Association.

Aronson, M.K., Post DC, Guastadisegni P. (1993). Dementia, Agitation, and Care in the Nursing Home. JAGS 41.

Ballard, C.G., O'Brien, J.T., Swann, A.G., Thompson P., Neill D., McKeith, I.G. (2001). The Natural History of Psychosis and Depression in Dementia with Lewy Bodies and Alzheimer's Disease: Persistance and New Cases Over One Year of Follow-Up. J. Clin. Psychiatry, 62.

Bear, D.M., Wolf, M.M., Todd, R., (1968). Some Current Dimensions of Applied Behavior Analysis. Journal of Applied Behavior Analysis.

Beard, R.M.F., (2001). Depression and Anxiety in Oncology: The Psychiatrist's Perspective. J. Clin. Psych. Suppl. 8.

Bellack, A.S., and Hersen, M., (1980). Introduction to Clinical Psychology. Behavior Therapy: Oxford University Press, New York, Oxford. 217-255.

Bensberg, G.J., and Sigelman, C.K., (1976). Definitions and Prevalence in L. L. Loyd Communication Assessment and Intervention Strategies. Baltimore University Park Press.

Burns, A., Jacoby, R. (1990). Psychiatric Phenomena in Alzheimer's Disease. 11: Disorders of Perception. British Journal of Psychiatry. 157.

Camp, C. J., and J. W. Foss. (1997). "Designing Ecologically Valid Memory Interventions for Persons with Dementia." In Intersections in Basic and Applied Memory Research, D. G. Payne and F. G. Conrad, eds. Hillsdale, NJ: Erlbaum.

Carstensen, L. L., Edelstein, B. A., and Dornbrand, L. (eds). (1966). The Practical Handbook of Clinical Gerontology. Thousand Oaks, CA: Sage.

Cohen, D., and Eisdorfer, C. (1993). Caring for your Aging Parents: A Planning and Action Guide. New York: Putnam.

Coleman, W.H., (2000). Importance of Behavioral and Psychological Symptoms of Dementia in Primary Care. International Psychogeriatrics, Vol. 12, Suppl. 1.

Costa, P.T., Jr., Williams, T.G., and Somerfield, M. (1996). "Recognition and Initial Assessment of Alzheimer's Disease and

Related Dementias." Clinical Practice Guideline, No. 19. Rockville, ND: Agency for Health Care Policy and Research, Public Health Service, U.S. Department of Health and Human Services.

Crosby, K.G., (1975). Essentials of Active Programming. Chicago: Joint Commission on Accreditation of Hospitals.

Cuccaro, E.F., Kramer, E., Zemishlany A., Thorne, A., Rice, M. et al. (1990). Pharmacologic treatment of Noncognitize Behavioral Disturbances in Elderly Demented Patients. A.M.J. Psychiatry Vol. 147.

Ditomasso, R.A., and Mills, O.F., (1990). The Behavioral Treatment of Essential Hypertension: Implications for Medical Psychotherapy. Medical Psychotherapy, An International Journal. Hogrefe and Huber Publishers, Inc., Toronto and New York. 125-134.

Doghramji, P.P., (2001). Detection of Insomnia in Primary Care. J. Clin. Psychiatry. Vol. 62. Suppl. 10.

Doka K., (2001). Challenging the Paradigm: New Understanding of Grief. The College of New Rochelle, New York.

Dwyther, L., (1987). "Traveling with the A.D. Patient: To Go or Not To Go?" The Caregiver Newsletter, Duke University.

Fein, N. (1993). The Validation Breakthrough: Simple Techniques for Communicating with People with Alzheimer's Type Dementia. Baltimore, MD: Health Professions Press.

Folsom, J. C., (1967). Attitude Therapy and the Team Approach. Faith at Work. October – November.

Folstein, J.F., Folstein, S.E., and McHugh, P.R., (1975). ."Mini-Mental State: A Practical Method for Grading the Cognitive State of Patients for the Clinician." Journal of Psychiatric Research, 12, 189-198.

Franks, C.M., (1969). Behavioral Therapy: Appraisal and Status. McGraw – Hill, New York.

Frazer, D.W., Jongsma, A.E., (1999). The Older Adult Psychotherapy, Treatment Planner: (Goals, Objectives, Therapeutic Interventions). John Wiley and Sons, Inc.

Friendland, R. P., Koss, E., Kumar, A., Gaine, S., Metzier D., Haxby, J. V., Moore A., (1988). Motor Vehicle Crashes in Dementia of the Alzheimer's Type, Ann. Neurol. Volume 24.

Gallagher, E., and Thompson, L. W., (1981). Depression in the Elderly: A Behavioral Treatment Manual. Los Angeles: The University of Southern California Press.

Gallagher, J. J., Surles, R. C., and Hayes, H. E., (1973). Program Planning and Evaluation. In First Chance for Children (Vol. 2). Frank Porter Graham Child Development Center, Chapel Hill, N.C.

Gilley, D., et al., (1991). Cessation of Driving and Unsafe Motor Vehicle Operation by Dementia Patients. Arch Intern. Med., Volume 15. May.

Guidance to Surveyors. Long Term Care Facilities (56 FR 48871, Sept. 26, 1991, as amended at 57 FR 43924), Sept. 23, 1992.

Hall, V. R. (1971). Managing Behavior. Part I. Behavior Modification: The Measurement of Behavior. H. and H. Enterprises. Lawrence, KS.

Hall, V. R. (1971). Managing Behavior. Part II. Behavior Modification: Basic Principles. H. and H. Enterprises. Lawrence, KS.

Hall, V. R. (1971). Managing Behavior. Part III. Behavior Modification: Applications in School and Home. H. and H. Enterprises. Lawrence, KS

Hall, V. R., Cristler, C., Bonnie, S. T., (1970). Teachers and Parents as Researchers Using Multiple Baseline Designs. Journal of Applied Behavior Analysis.

Hartman-Stein, P.E. (ed,) (1988). Innovative Behavioral Healthcare for Older Adults: A Guidebook for Changing Tiems. San Francisco: Jossey-Bass.

Hensley, G., and Patterson, V. (1970). Interdisciplinary Programming for Infants with Known or Suspected Cerebral Dysfunctional. Boulder, DO: Western Interstate Commission for Higher Education.

Houts, P. S., and Scott, R. A., (1975). Goal Planning with Developmentally Disabled Persons. Hershey, PA.: The Commonwealth of Pennsylvania.

Hussian, R. A., and Davis, R. L., (1985). Responsive Care: Behavioral Interventions with Elderly Persons. Champaign, IL: Research Press.

Israel, S. A., (2000). Insomnia in the Elderly: A Review for the Primary Care Practitioner. Sleep, Vol. 23, Suppl. 1.

Jongsma, Q. E., Peterson, L. M., McInnis, W. P., (1996). The Child and Adolescent Psychotherapy; Treatment Planner. (Behavior Definitions, Long Term Goals, Short Term Objectives, Therapeutic Interventions). John Wiley and Sons, Inc. New York.

Kane, R. A., and Caplan, A. L., (eds.). (1990). Everyday Ethics: Resolving Dilemmas in Nursing Home Life. New York: Springer.

Klerman, G. L., Budman, S., Berwick, D., Weissman, M. M., Damico-White, J., Demby, A., and Feldstein, M., (1987). "Efficacy of a Brief Psychosocial Intervention for Symptoms of Stress and Distress Among Patients in Primary Care." Medical Care, 25, 1078-1088.

Knight, B. G. (1996). Psychotherapy with Older Adults, 1 nd ed. Boston: Allyn and Bacon.

Kunik, M. E., Yudofsky, S. C., Silver, J. M., Hales, R. E. (1994). Pharmacologic Approach to Management of Agitation Associated with Dementia. J. Clin. Psychiatry. Vol. 55, Suppl. 2.

LaRue, A. (1992). Aging and Neuropsychological Assessment. New York: Plenum.

Laughren T. Regulatory, (2000). Issues on Behavioral and Psychological Symptoms of Dementia in the United States. International Psychogeriatrics, Vol. 12, Suppl. 1.

Laurin, D., Verreault, R., Lindsay, J., MacPherson, K., Rockwood, K (2001). Physical Activity and Risk of Cognitive Impairment and Dementia in Elderly Persona. Arch. Neurol. Vol. 58.

Lawton, M. P., and Brody, E. M., (1969). "Assessment of Older People: Self-Maintaining and Instrumental Activities of Daily Living." The Gerontologist, 9, 179-185.

Lent, J. R., and Keilitz, I., (1974). How to do More: A Manual of Basic Teaching Strategies. Belview, WA: Edmark Associates.

Levey, D. T., Vernick, T. S., Howard, K. A., (1995). Relationships Between Driver's License Renewal Policies and Fatal Crashes Involving Drivers 70 Years or Older, JAMA, October. No. 13, Volume 274.

Levy, M. I., Cummings, J. L., Fairbanks, L. A., Bravi, D., Calvani, M., Carta, A., (1996), Longitudinal Assessment of Symptoms of Depression, Agitation, and Psychosis in 181 Patients with Alzheimer's Diseases: Am. J. Psychiatry. 153.

Lichtenberg, P. A., (1994). A Guide to Psychological Practice in

Geriatric Long Term Care. Binghamton, NY: Haworth Press.
Lichtenberg, P. A.,a nd Strzepek, D. M., (1990). "Assessments of
Institutionalized Dementia Patients' Competencies to Participate in
Intimate Relationships." The Gerontologist, 30, 117-120.

Lichtenberg, P. A., Smith, M., Frazer, D., Molinari, V., Rosowsky,
R., Crose, R., Stillwell, N., Kramer, N., Hartman-Stein, P., Qualls,
S., Salamon, M., Duffy, M., Parr, J., and Gallagher-Thompson, D.,
(1998). "Standards for Psychological Services in Long-Term Care
Facilities." The Gerontologist, 38(1), 122-127.

Lyketsos, C. G., Steele, C., Galik, E., Rosenblatt, A., Steinberg,
M., Warren, A., Sheppard, J. M., (1999). Physical Aggression
in Dementia Patients and Its Relationship to Depression. Am. J.
Psychiatry. Vol. 156.

Mace, N. L., and Rabins, P. V., (1991). The Thirty-Six-Hour Day: A
Family Guide to Caring for Persons with Alzheimer's Disease, Related
Dementing Illnesses, and Memory Loss in Later Life. Baltimore,
MD: Johns Hopkins University Press.

Mager, R. F., (1961). Preparing Instructional Objectives. Fearon
Publishers, Belmont, CA.

Maurer, T.A., (2002). Alzheimer's Care: Combining High – Tech
with High – Touch. Responses to an Aging Florida. Atlanta.

McCurry, S. M., Logsdon, R. G., Vitiello, M. V., and Terri, L.,
(1998). "Successful Behavioral Treatment for Reported Sleep
Problems in Elderly Caregivers of Dementia Patients: A Controlled
Study." Journal of Gerontology: Psychological Sciences, 53B, P122-
P129.

McShane, R., (2000). What are the Syndromes of Behavioral
and Psychological Symptoms of Dementia? International
Psychogeriatrics, Vol. 12, Suppl. L.

Migiacclo, J. N., (2002). Assisted Living Today: Vol. 9, No. 5. Advanced Monitoring Systems Provide Clules to Resident Challenges, Enabling Staff to Provide Better Care. NY

Morrison, J., (1995). DSM-IV Made Easy: Delirium, Dementia, and Amnestic and Other Cognitive Disorders. New York, London: The Guilford Press.

Minimum Standards of Operation for Alzheimer's Disease/Dementia Care Unit (2001). Ms. St. Dept. of Health. Health Facilities Licensure and Certification, Post Office Box 1700, Jackson, MS 39215-1700.

Nathan, P. E., and Gorman, J . M., (eds.). (1998). A Guide to Treatments That Work. New York: Oxford.

National Center for Cost Containment. (1997). Assessment of Competency and Capacity of the Older Adult: A Practice Guideline for Psychologists. Washington, D. C.: U. S. Department of Veterans Affairs.

National Center for Cost Containment. (1996). Geropsychology Assessment Resource Guide. Washington, D. C.: U. S. Department of Veterans Affairs (PB-96-144365).

Parmelee, P. A., Katz, I. R., Lawton, M. P., (1992). Incidence of Depression in Long-Term Care Settings. Journal of Gerontology Medical Sciences. Vol. 47, No. 6.

Petersen, R. C., Smith, G. E., Waring S. C., Ivnik, R. J., Tangalos, E. G., Kokmen, E., (1999). Mild Cognitive Impairment; Clinical Characterization and Outcome. Arch. Neurol. Vol. 56.

Poon, L., Crook, T., Davis, K., Eisdorfer, C., Gurland, B., Kaszniak, A., and Thompson, L. W., (eds.) (1989). Handbook for Clinical Memory Assessment of Older Adults. Washington, D. C.: American

Psychological Association.

Powers, R. E. (2003). Bridging the Continuum of Care: DETA Training. Alzheimer's Conference. The University of Alabama, Tuscaloosa, AL.

Ramage, J. W., (1971). The Problem of Mental Health. Nursing Homes. Vol. 20, No. 5.

Raskin, A., and Niederehe, G., (eds.) (1988). "Assessment in Diagnosis and Treatment of Geropsychiatric Patients." Psychopharmacology Bulletin (Special Feature), DHHS Publication No. (ADM) 88-173. Rockville, MD: Department of Health and Human Services, 24(4).

Reisberg, B., Borenstein, J., Franssen, E., Shulman, E., Steinberg, G., Ferris, S. H., (1986). Remediable Behavioral Symptomatology in Alzheimer's Disease. Hospital and Community Psychiatry. Vol. 37, No. 12.

Rheume, Y. "Wandering", Dementia Study Unit, Veterans Administration Hospital, Bedford, MA.

Ritchie, K., Artero, S., Touchon, J., (2001). Classification Criteria for Mild Cognitive Impairment: A Population-Based Validation Study. Neurology, Vol. 56.

Robinson, A., Spencer, B., and White, L., (1991). "Understanding Difficult Behaviors: Some Practical Suggestions for Coping with Alzheimer's Disease and Related Illness." Geriatric Education Center of Michigan.

Rubin, D. B., (1991). Dementia and Driving. Journal of the American Geriatrics Society, Vol. 39. Number 11. November.

Schneider, L. S., (1996). Overview of Generalized Anxiety Disorder in the Elderly. J. Clin. Psychiatry. Suppl. 7.

Schulberg, H. C., Alan, S., and Frank, B., (1969). Program Evaluation in the Health Field. Behavioral Publishers, New York.

Schulz, I. L., and Texidor, M. S., (1991). The Interdisciplinary Approach: An Exercise in Futility or a Song of Praise: Medical Psychotherapy, An International Journal. Hogrefe and Huber Publishers, Inc. Toronto and New York. 1-8.

Schwartz, R., (2003). Update on Alzheimer's Disease Fourth Annual Conference on Alzheimer's Disease and Psychiatric Disorders in the Elderly. Philadelphia, MS.

Scott, W. G., (1961). Organizational Theory: An Overview and an Appraisal. Journal of the Academy of Management.

Seldes, George., (1985). The Great Thoughts. Ballantine Books. New York.

Sheikh, J. I., (1991). "Anxiety Rating Scales for the Elderly." In Anxiety in the Elderly: Treatment and Research, Salzman, D., and Lebowitz, B. D. (eds.) New York: Springer Publishing.

Sheikh, J. I., and Yesavage, J. A., (1986). "Geriatric Depression Scale (GDS): Recent Evidence and Development of a Shorter Version." Clinical Gerontologist, 5, 165-173.

Shuster, J. L., (2000). Palliative Care for Advanced Dementia: Death and Dying. Clinics in Geriatric Medicine. Vol. 16.

Skinner, B. F., (1953). Science and Human Behavior. New York: MacMillan Co.

Small, G. W., Hormone Treatments for Behavioral and Psychological Symptoms of Dementia. International Psychogeriatrics, Vol. 12, Suppl. 1.

Small, S. Q., (2001). Age-Related Memory Decline. Current Concepts and Future Directions. ARCH. Neurol. Vol. 58.

Souder, E., Heithoff, K., O'Sullivan, P. S., Lancaster, A.E., Beck, C., (1999). Identifying Patterns of Disruptive Behavior in Long-Term Care Residents. JAGS 47.

Stern, L., and Fogler, J., (1988). Improving Your Memory: A Guide for Older Adults. Ann Arbor, MI: Memory Skills.

Sze, W. C., and Hopps, J. G., (1974). Evaluation and Accountability in Human Service Programs. Schenkman Publishing Co., Cambridge, MA.

Teri, L., et al., (1994). Aging and Dementia: Reducing Disability in Alzheimer's Disease. A Manual for Therapists. Seattle, WA: University of Washington.

Teri, L., and Gallaghes, D., (1991). "Cognitive Behavior Interventions for Treatment of Depression." The Gerontologist, 31, 413-416.

Teri, L., and Logsdon, R., (1991). Identifying Pleasant Activities for Alzheimer's Disease Patients: The Pleasant Events Schedule – AD. The Gerontologist, 31, 124-127.

Trobe, J. D., Waller, P. F., Flanagan, C. A., Teshima, S. M., Crashes and Violations Among Drivers with Alzheimer's Disease, (1996). ARCH Neurol. Vol 53, May.

U. S. Department of Health and Human Services, Office of the Inspector General, (1996). Mental Health Services in Nursing Facilities. Washington, D. C.: U. S. Department of Health and Human Services.

U. S. Department of Veterans Affairs and University Health System

Consortium., (1997). Dementia Identification and Assessment: Guidelines for Primary Care Practitioners. Washington, D. C.: U. S. Department of Veterans Affairs.

Wisocki, P. A. (ed.). Handbook of Clinical Behavior Therapy with the Elderly Client. New York: Plenum.

Worden, W., (1991). Grief Counseling and Grief Therapy, 2nd ed. New York: Springer.

Yesavage, J. A., Brink, T. L., and Rose, T. L., (1983). "Development and Validation of a Geriatric Depression Scale: A Preliminary Report, Journal of Psychiatric Residents, 17, 37-49.

Yesavage, J. A., Brink, T. L., Rose, T., and Adey, M., (1983). "The Geriatric Depression Scale: Comparison with Other Self-Report and Psychiatric Rating Scales. In Assessment in Geriatric Psychopharmacology, Crook, T., Ferris, S., and Bahrs, R., eds. New Canaan, CT: Mark Pouley Associates, 152-167.

Zubenko, G. S., (2000). Neurobiology of Major Depression in Alzheimer's Disease. International Psychiatrics, Vol. 12, Suppl. 1.

AFTERWORD

This author has presented a model of an Individual Therapeutic Activity Plan (ITAP). It contains four basic parts: 1) goals, 2) objectives, 3) strategies, and 4) evaluation. As you, the reader, become more familiar and increasingly skillful with the procedures for writing an ITAP, you may want to adapt this basic model to suit your own needs or develop your own. However, whatever the case, there are some basic principles of an ITAP which remain constant. For example, they are written by an interdisciplinary team for every resident accepted for services. They include both long-term goals and objectives; are reviewed at least annually, and involve the resident, family, and his or her advocate to the fullest extent possible as a member of the treatment team. The forms included in this book are merely examples of how an ITAP might be written, and is in no way intended to interfere with your creativity and imagination in developing your own.

Each ITAP is individualized because that is the only way to assure that each resident who participates in a training program will have a plan especially designed to meet his or her own specific needs. This kind of planning for residents demand your greatest sensitivity and motivation. As you work to implement an ITAP, there are times when you as a trainer may become frustrated and would like to regress back into the habit of generalizing about the resident(s) who are difficult. However, if you develop and write your ITAP(s) consistently and approach your training as carefully as you plan, you will find resident achievements excel where you expected none. You will be giving your residents the best opportunity to maintain and or increase their skills and improve their quality of life.

And in conclusion, nothing in this book is intended to constitute medical or professional treatment, specific prescription or advice. Medical diagnosis and treatment can only occur between an individual and his or her physician.

ABOUT THE AUTHOR

Dr. Ramage, is currently a psychotherapist, in private practice specializing in Gerontology. He holds degrees in both clinical social work and behavioral psychology. He is a diplomate in clinical social work, a fellow and diplomate in medical psychotherapy, and is an activity consultant certified with the National Certification Council for Activity Professionals. He is listed in Who's Who in the American Academy of Human Services and in Who's Who Among Human Service Professionals.

A life – long student of human behavior, Dr. Ramage received his undergraduate degree at Delta State University. His graduate training was completed at the University of Tennessee, Florida State, and Walden Universities. He interned in the Departments of Psychiatry at Vanderbilt University Hospital in Nashville, The University of Mississippi Medical Center in Jackson, and The University of North Carolina at Chapel Hill. As an intern, he was privileged to be a student of the renowned Psychiatrist, Author and Lecturer, Dr. Viktor Frankl, Psychiatrists Drs. Joe D. Woddail and James C. Folsom, of the Menninger Clinic, and a noted social worker, author, Family Therapist and Lecturer, Dr. Virginia Satir.

Dr. Ramage, ACSW, LCSW, PIP, ACC is presently CEO of Associated Healthcare Consultants, a company he founded in 1970 to address the psychological needs of nursing home residents and their families. The philosophy which Dr. Ramage brought to the company was to provide a program of services which adhered to a team approach, continuity of care and to the basic principles of behavior modification. He mandated that all activity plans be developed by an interdisciplinary team and contain four basic elements of service: 1) goals, 2) objectives, 3) strategies and 4) evaluation, a program procedure now required in most nursing home facilities by Federal and State Regulatory Agencies.

www.ingramcontent.com/pod-product-compliance
Lightning Source LLC
Chambersburg PA
CBHW031824170526
45157CB00001B/177